NUTRITION, HEALTH & DISEASE

D1407914

NUTRITION, HEALTH & DISEASE

GARY PRICE TODD, M.D.

FOREWORD BY ELMER CRANTON, M.D.

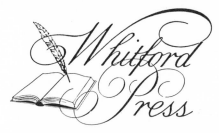

A division of Schiffer Publishing, Ltd.
1469 Morstein Road
West Chester, Pennsylvania 19380 USA

Distributed by Schiffer Publishing, Ltd.
1469 Morstein Road
West Chester, Pennsylania 19380
Please write for a free catalog
This book may be purchased from the publisher.
Please include $2.00 postage.
Try your bookstore first.

Library of Congress Cataloging in Publication Data

Todd, Gary Price.
  Nutrition, health, and disease.

  Bibliography: p
  Includes index.
    1. Health   2. Nutrition.   3. Deficiency diseases.   4. Holistic medicine.
I. Title. (DNLM: 1. Health.   2. Nutrition—popular works. QU 145 T634n)
RA784.T63   1985   616.3'9   85-10215
ISBN: 0-89865-404-1 (pbk.)

Printed in the United States of America

Table of Contents

Preface

Dr. Todd and I share a common interest in nutrition. We both developed our interest in nutritional medicine along a common pathway. A series of events in our professional lives penetrated a strong bias against nutrition, the result of a traditional medical education, and directed our energies toward this neglected but extremely important aspect of health care. In my case, it was the observation that patients in my practice, who had obtained nutritional advice elsewhere, seemed to benefit from that advice, despite my expectation to the contrary.

I then devoted a large portion of my free time to an independent search of the scientific literature concerning nutrition and preventive medicine. I was amazed to find a very large body of research and well documented scientific knowledge which had been completely ignored in my curriculum at Harvard Medical School. As I increasingly applied these principles in my practice, health benefits were observed which I had not previously believed possible. More recently, I have become interested in free radical pathology, an important common denominator of both Dr. Todd's work and mine.

Although the final answers concerning nutrition and free radical pathology are not yet known, Dr. Todd's discoveries and observations described in this book have a sound scientific basis. There is a growing body of evidence that supports his thesis that our diet does not supply enough nutrients for optimum health. In fact, the evidence is overwhelming that even the most carefully planned diet is less than adequate, and that significant benefits can be obtained at modest cost with the addition of nutritional supplements.

Although this book presents material that has been known for some years, it is unique and well worth study by those who wish to enjoy optimum health. It is a book to be read, reread, and digested. Yes, and enjoyed; for enjoy you will. The wealth of information contained within these pages could very well save your life. The chapters on weight control, vision, cholesterol, and cancer are especially incisive, and include information which would be difficult to find elsewhere. All in all, this work integrates a tremendous amount of information into an intelligent and concise form. It is not the final answer in nutrition; but it can open your eyes to a need, and point you in directions where your needs can be met.

Both Dr. Todd and I agree that there is more to life than is visible to the eye, and that healing involves more than just medicine or nutrition. The most effective physician will be one who combines traditional medicine with nutrition and preventive principles, within a framework of strong spiritual values, and with proper consideration for the mental and emotional aspects of health. This, in the truest sense, is what holistic medicine is all about. Good medicine is holistic medicine! It always has been, and it always will be.

Elmer M. Cranton, M.D.
Mount Rogers Clinic
Trout Dale, Virginia

Note:

Dr. Elmer M. Cranton is past president of the American Holistic Medical Association and past president of the Smyth County Medical Society, Virginia. He is a board certified specialist in both Family Practice and Chelation Therapy, and currently serves as executive vice president of the American Academy of Medical Preventics. Dr. Cranton has authored two books which are currently in print: *Trace Elements, Hair Analysis and Nutrition,* and *By-Passing Bypass—The New Techniques of Chelation Therapy.*

Introduction

After years of experience in nutritional therapy, I firmly believe that the average American diet is woefully deficient. And worse, there is mounting evidence that it is impossible to devise a diet that provides optimal health.

Three factors have made an ideal diet nearly impossible. First, the deteriorated state of our soils due to erosion, pesticides, and overuse of chemical fertilizers. Second, many dietary molecules are modified by food processors so that they no longer are beneficial but are actually toxic when consumed. Third, many nutrients and trace elements are removed or lost from foods during processing, storage, and preparation.

Obviously, our diet is capable to sustaining life for the traditional threescore and ten. Optimum health, on the other hand, could possibly result in a lifespan well over a century, perhaps even the biblical promise of 120 years.

I am convinced that everyone must become increasingly responsible for his own health. Our economy cannot afford a population dependent upon health care professionals for every facet of their care, nor will it be possible to train sufficient numbers of qualified professionals to treat such a dependent population. Good nutrition would greatly reduce the frequency of illness and the cost of health care, which would solve both problems.

Anytime an author takes pen in hand to put down in black and white those thoughts he feels useful to others, he is building upon the works and genius of his contemporaries and predecessors. Just as gold is where you find it, I have freely accepted knowledge from others, regardless of their formal qualifications. I do, however, owe a special debt to certain special people: my wife, Clara, and my two sons, Frank and George, who have had to put up with my eccentricities and absence necessitated by the writing of this book; and to those regional physicians who have supported me in my efforts to alert our patients and friends to the need for better nutrition. Several physicians have taken their time to read and critically review the manuscript in its various stages of completion.

They have given precious time and effort to another's work, and that sacrifice is greatly appreciated. Included in this group are Dr. Elmer M. Cranton, an author and leader in nutritional and chelation therapy research; Dr. Harry H. Summerlin, Jr., a physician in family practice, who, like myself, is active in the Boy Scout movement; and Dr. Logan Robertson, a close friend and physician in the true sense of the word. Dr. H. Dwight Cavanagh, the chairman of the Department of Ophthalmology at Emory University has given of his time and advice. Dr. Robert Cooper, Chief of Hematology and Oncology at The Bowman Grey School of Medicine, has reviewed this manuscript and given his moral and constructive support to this effort. I am deeply indebted to each of these men's suggestions and sacrifice.

Carefully evaluate what I have included in this book and tailor it to your own situation. Find other books written by those professionals with nutritional experience and study them. Your life and health will be greatly rewarded.

It is necessary, because of FDA bias, to make a disclaimer at this point: this book is not designed to eliminate personal professional consultation, nor are the concepts intended to be used in any specific situation without consultation with someone who is knowledgeable in medicine and nutritional concepts. This book is intended to open the mind of the reader to a need so that intelligent decisions might be made, affecting the reader's health and life.

I do not wish to lay at the feet of any of the above named scholars the burden of defending what I have written. I take full personal responsibility for what I have written. Time will confirm much of what is in this book. Time will also prove a lot of it to be in error. I have tried to make it as current as possible, completely revising the book three times as new information became available. My hope is that this book has sufficient impact to force additional research in these areas, and thereby prove to have been worth my effort.

Gary Price Todd, MD
112 Academy Street
Waynesville, NC USA
(704) 456-3506

Foreword

Nutrition is an ongoing science. What is thought to be right in 1987 may not be proper in 1990 or the year 2000. What Dr. Gary Todd has done is to follow through with his use of nutritional supplements with his cataract patients. Under this regime approximately 50% had an increase of vision to a useful level. In America that is a breakthrough. Most of the cataract patients seen by the eye specialists should be given a three to six-month trial with an appropriate nutritional product that is rich in glutathione, also antioxidants such as ascorbic acid, vitamin E, zinc, beta carotene and selenium. If still indicated in three to six months then do cataract surgery. My studies reveal hundreds of European articles on the medical treatment of cataracts with about the same 50% rate of reversal as shown by Dr. Todd. Several double-blind controlled studies done there confirm these rates of increased vision.

We are looking forward at the Biomedical Research Institute of America of having Dr. Gary Todd become a fellow researcher. Although he may still be in North Carolina we will do what we can to help in his studies and the publication of the resulting research articles.

I predict when competent eye specialists in this country get into the nonsurgical treatment of cataracts that there will be fewer and fewer cataracts that need surgery.

Other ocular diseases which are responding to nutritional therapy include macular degeneration, glaucoma, diabetic retinopathy, and dry eye syndrome. This is indeed a fertile field for research, as witnessed by the tremendous number of research articles worldwide on the effect of nutrition on vision.

Are there other eye problems that might respond to nutritional supplements? We can't say but we hope to have more facts soon. Good luck in your future studies Gary.

—Bruce A. Sanderson, M.D.

Bruce A. Sanderson, M.D., is a past president of the Biochemical Research Institute of America, and a current board member. He is currently an Adjunct Professor of the School of Medicine of the Loma Linda University, and past Chief of Otolaryngology. He is still active in research, and has a special interest in nutrition as it applies to vision.

I.
A Primer in Nutrition

From the day you were born until today, every molecule within your body got there by being eaten. A purist may argue that some molecules got in by other means; but with rare exceptions, we are what we eat. These molecules have definite purposes, and are absolutely necessary for life and good health. Some are required in extremely small quantities, so small that the weight of the period at the end of this sentence far exceeds the weight needed. Other minerals are needed in relatively large quantities, measured in thousands of grams daily. Therefore, do not be deceived into believing that good nutrition is not important, nor that it comes automatically with three meals a day. It is important, but it does not come automatically.

Your body needs six classes of substances in order to remain healthy. These are proteins, carbohydrates, fats, minerals, fiber, and vitamins.

Proteins are made up of approximately twenty amino acids, the building blocks of any protein molecule. Of these twenty amino acids found in the body, your body can synthesize all but nine. These nine are essential amino acids and *all* must be present in *each* meal in the right proportions, otherwise the rest of the amino acids cannot be used to make protein, and are converted to glucose or fat. Think of amino acids as pieces of a puzzle. If even one piece of the puzzle is missing, then the whole puzzle is thrown away as worthless. Your body is a little more conservative, and rather than throwing it away, converts the extra amino acids to sources of energy. Beef and milk have the proper mix of amino acids, and are considered to be high quality proteins. Most cereal grains are deficient in one or more amino acids, and therefore much of the protein from cereal grains (corn, wheat, barley, rye, and so forth) is not used as protein, but is converted to energy. Fortunately, the amino acid deficiency is different for different vegetables, so that eating a variety of vegetables can provide an

1

adequate mixture of essential amino acids. The most common amino acid deficiency in cereals is lysine. Soybeans are rich in lysine, but are poor in methionine. Soybean protein is therefore a good supplement when eaten with a meal with other cereal grains. Some soybean protein food supplements have been augmented with methionine, so that its efficiency is two and one-half times that of usual dietary protein. The poor quality of the average vegetable protein eaten in America would require 75 grams daily to meet recommended daily allowances. It only takes 45 grams of high quality protein, such as is in beef or milk, or in an augmented soybean protein to meet your daily needs. Limiting your consumption of protein to that actually needed is not only cheaper, but reduces the amount of by-products which must be purged by the kidneys.

For most Americans, the quantity of protein eaten daily is far in excess of that needed. Even worse, our preferred sources of protein are also rich in peroxidized fats and sodium, and poor in potassium. We would be much healthier to reduce our intake of red meat to about four ounces per day, or even less, and supplement our diet with soybean protein. If you are a vegetarian, then an augmented soybean protein is ideal, because it is a complete protein and would supply all your protein needs with two servings daily. Vegetarian diets are generally deficient in quality protein, especially the amino acid lysine. However, vegetarians are generally healthier than those whose diet is centered on meat. Because vegetables (unless smothered in butter) are lower in calories than meat products, vegetarians are less likely to be overweight or to suffer from those diseases associated with obesity. Additionally, there is experimental evidence to support the contention that a diet relatively deficient in calories, but rich in vitamins and trace nutrients, contributes to a longer (and healthier) lifespan.

Although protein deficiency is a problem in Third World nations, it is definitely not a problem in the United States. Our problem is that we get too many of our calories from meat (and the fat in meat), and thus neglect vegetable sources of calories. The vegetables contain necessary vitamins, minerals, and fiber not found in meat. The average American eats a "meat and potatoes" diet. Not that these are not good, wholesome foods: they are. But this is decidedly not a balanced diet, and we should not pretend it is.

My main admonition concerning protein is to eat only enough meat to supply about 30 grams of protein daily. This will mean only about four ounces of lean meat daily. The rest of your protein

2

should come from vegetable sources. Of these, the soybean protein to which methionine has been added is clearly superior. You can grow soybeans in your garden; and if picked when the beans are full but still green, they can be served like lima beans. Mixed with another source of vegetable protein (beans, corn, wheat), they have a nutitional value similar to meat. I believe soybeans, eaten with another protein-rich vegetable, should be included frequently in your diet. I prefer the taste of soybeans to other garden beans because they taste a lot like boiled peanuts, a favorite of mine. So much for my Southern ancestry.

The rest of your calories should be made up with vegetables. The fat you need will come almost automatically. I do not agree with those who insist that the fats in the diet should be all unsaturated. Unsaturated fats are unstable, and deteriorate on exposure to oxygen (in the air) to produce some very toxic compounds. These toxic compounds are combated in the body by producing cholesterol, which is a potent antioxidant, or with dietary antioxidants such as the beta carotenes (provitamin A), the vitamins niacin, riboflavin, C and E and the minerals manganese, selenium, and zinc. Oxidation of oils outside the body can be slowed by use of antioxidants; but unfortunately, the use of antioxidants is unpopular among advocates of health food today, so food processors have stopped using these valuable products as a result of the bad press. Remember, while these preservatives are preserving the food, they are also preserving you. You would be a lot safer to use butter than to switch to liquid oils which cannot be kept fresh. Just recently a report was released linking the increase in stomach cancer in the U.S. to the use of cooking oils for cooking French fries in fast food restaurants, probably the major source of peroxidized fats in the American diet today. There have been studies that clearly show that butter will not produce carcinogens (cancer-causing compounds) during frying, while unsaturated oils commonly produce carcinogens. This is because saturated fats, such as butter, do not readily oxidize into toxic lipid peroxides, whereas unsaturated fats do. *If you re-use your cooking oils, you are greatly compounding your risk.* Current medical thinking is that unsaturated fats are necessary to reduce blood cholesterol, but there are better ways to cut cholesterol without the risk of rancid oils.

Like your body, plants get their trace elements from their diet. Therefore, the elements in vegetables can only be those which are present in the soil. That is, if the elements are missing in the soil, they will be missing in the vegetables. Most unfortunately, vegetables can thrive without many elements needed by us, and if

3

these elements are missing they do not end up in the vegetables we eat. Modern farming methods generally only add the minerals necessary for the vegetables to grow, and ignore that the purpose of growing the vegetables should be to produce healthy humans. Therefore, the farmer usually only adds nitrogen, potassium, and phosphorus to the soil. Calcium and magnesium are also added periodically to control soil acidity. With time, the other elements are gradually lost from the soil, unless organic techniques are followed to add back these trace elements. This is well known to occur with grass, so that cattle will die unless the needed elements are added through the use of mineral salts. I suspect that the only reason we are not dying with severe trace element deficiencies is that we eat enough beef to offset the deficiencies found in our vegetables. The cattle get theirs from the mineral salts they eat.

Trace element deficiencies are very common in America. In fact, the Senate Select Committee on Nutrition concluded that 99 percent of Americans suffer from mineral deficiencies. The chances that your diet contains the recommended dietary allowance of major trace elements is really very slim. Once you realize that your diet *may* be deficient, your mind is open to analysing your diet and correcting the deficiencies. As long as you believe the myth of the perfect American diet, you run the risk of poor health due to deficiencies. That risk is close to 100 percent.

The best solution to the problem is to have a good garden plot, and enrich the soil with mulch from leaves and any organic scraps you can find. Green sand, a product of the sea, is rich in minerals and will supply the trace elements we need. Some farmers also use seaweed and kelp to add trace elements.

If you can't do that, then you will have to supplement your diet with trace elements. The best sources will be ocean salt (used sparingly), seafoods both animal and vegetable, and alfalfa. More expensive, but very effective sources, are yeasts that have been grown on broths rich in those elements. Unfortunately, yeasts have a high potential for allergic reactions, perhaps because so many of us are sensitized by Candida albicans overgrowth. Spirulina is the best example of a natural algae product rich in trace elements. Mineral supplement tablets are available, but will only have those elements currently recognized, if those. Only within the past year have the importance of selenium and chromium been recognized, and few products available contain these in adequate quantities. It has been at least three years since zinc deficiency was proven to be common, and many mineral supplements still do not contain adequate amounts of zinc. Undoubtedly, other elements will prove to be essential to good health, even in extremely small quantities. We are, after all, made of clay. The best way to guarantee that you will get enough of these elements is to use natural sources which are grown in soil (or in the sea) rich in all elements. The value of seafoods is obvious. Alfalfa is less obviously of value, but is most valuable because its roots go deep within the earth, penetrating to a depth of over forty feet. Thus the alfalfa leaves have elements long since lost to the topsoil, and not present in most garden vegetables. It is possibly these trace elements that make alfalfa leaves so effective in promoting growth in garden vegetables, when used as a mulch, and in animals when used as food.

Soil erosion has depleted the vast majority of topsoil present when we began farming this continent a century ago. Intensive chemical fertilizers have kept crop production up, but the essential trace and major element content of our crops has decreased markedly. Among those elements commonly deficient in vegetables grown with commercial fertilizers are chromium, magnesium, manganese, selenium, vanadium, and zinc. Consistent use of pesticides has resulted in an almost sterile soil, reducing action by bacteria and earthworms which would release micronutrients for use by plants, and eventually by us. Topsoil is not just the top few inches of dirt, it is alive. That topsoil is alive is not overstating the facts, it is perhaps understating an urgent reality we must learn to protect. All life on earth depends on the health of the top eight inches of soil, and the top few hundred feet of ocean. To lose sight of that is to suffer severely. This is the best argument in favor of environmental issues and diet supplementation today. Unless you grow your own vegetables and know that the soil has ample trace elements, do not depend on your diet supplying these without supplements.

Two such (former) deficiencies are now widely recognized, and as a result iron and iodine are added to commonly eaten foods. It is unlikely that deficiencies of these two minerals will occur except rarely. In fact, supplementation of these two elements is so extensive that most Americans are ingesting potentially toxic amounts of iron, and many times the amount of iodine needed. Other deficiencies are also common, but unrecognized, so that almost everyone suffers from them. At least 80 percent of those whom I have questioned have a diet deficient in calcium according to the RDA, and studies clearly indicate zinc deficiency in perhaps 85 percent of the population. Chromium and selenium deficiencies are almost universal, except in areas such as Nebraska where ancient volcanic activity has left the soil very rich in selenium.

5

Almost everyone gets many times the sodium needed, so that the ratio of potassium to sodium is grossly distorted. This is the result of our high meat, low vegetable diet. Meat is high in sodium, while vegetables are high in potassium. (However, most canned vegetables are prepared with salt, and are thus often high in sodium.)

Within the past several decades, several major changes have occurred in the American diet. We have switched from a high vegetable to a high meat diet. Salt has become cheap and plentiful, and is used extensively to enhance the flavor of canned and processed foods. These two factors have resulted in a switch from a high potassium, low sodium diet, to the present high sodium, relatively low potassium diet. This has upset the important potassium/sodium ratio so necessary for good health. Our bread is now processed to remove the bran and germ so that it will store without spoiling. In fact, it is so devoid of nutritional value that even insects cannot live on the stuff. Because our soils are depleted, our vegetables no longer are a good source of elements other than calcium, potassium, phosphorus, and magnesium. Canning foods has resulted in a high loss of the many heat sensitive vitamins such as B-complex, C and E. We have increasingly turned to highly processed foods such as potato chips and carbonated beverages which are totally devoid of any nutrition other than calories, and are also high in sodium and phosphorus. Carbonated beverages are high in phosporic acid, added to control acidity (and to dissolve the cola), which binds dietary calcium and further depletes the body of needed calcium.

Some of our well-intentioned plans have gone awry. Chlorine added to purify our water supply destroys vitamin E, and has been proven to be a cause of atherosclerosis, at least in chickens. I have absolutely no doubt that chlorinated water is a cause of atherosclerosis and other degenerative diseases. Unsaturated fats added to the diet to reduce cholesterol also require a higher dietary intake of vitamin E to protect them from peroxidation, but we have decreased our intake of vitamin E through the use of bleached flour and hot pressing our oils. (Even worse, oil processors remove the commercially valuable vitamin E for sale separately.) The list is endless. The result is an epidemic of degenerative diseases unheard of at the turn of the century.

Carbohydrates are another major food group that we all seem to get in sufficient quantity, but not in the right quality. Carbohydrates are a major source of energy, in fact the only form of food that can be used directly as energy. Carbohydrates can be simple, such as sugar; or complex, such as cellulose. Starch is intermediate in complexity. Human beings cannot digest cellulose, so cellulose forms the bulk of fiber in our diets. The body converts all other carbohydrates to glucose, also known as dextrose, before using them for energy. Glucose is converted back to complex carbohydrates for storage as glycogen, or converted to fats for storage as fat. Both fat and protein (amino acids) can be converted to glucose for energy. The human body is designed for a diet in which the major component is complex carbohydrates. Complex carbohydrates result in a more stable blood sugar. This effect may be more due to trace elements present in unprocessed vegetables and grains than to the complex carbohydrates themselves, but this is a question as yet unsettled. The modern diet, however, has shifted from complex carbohydrates such as found in vegetables, to simple carbohydrates such as sugar. Almost all prepared foods have very high proportions of sugar, and in addition to sugar use carbohydrates such as starch which are intermediate in complexity. The result is an epidemic of high and low blood sugar which has been recognized within the past decade. The carbohydrates in our modern diet are digested too quickly for the body to move them into storage forms. As a result our blood sugar shoots too high shortly after a meal of junk food, and overcorrects to a low blood sugar about one hour later. The result is a feeling of exhaustion about an hour after a meal. This epidemic is so common that even the general public recognizes the term hypoglycemia. Certain vitamins and minerals are needed to metabolize carbohydrates, and these are also commonly deficient in processed foods, but are present in natural carbohydrate rich foods.

However, the absence of micronutrients is not the entire answer, because sugar, antibiotics, steroids, and birth control pills all stimulate the overgrowth of the yeast, Candida albicans. When further stimulated by sugar, the yeast in our gut releases over sixty substances which are either toxic, endocrine active, or allergenic substances. Thus, our poor diet plus drug useage leads to yeast overgrowth, which in turn produces a multiplicity of allergic and abnormal reactions to food. This concept is far from academic: I know of one lady who finally found her way to Dr. Logan Robertson, who diagnosed her many food allergies as the result of Candidiasis, and treated her appropriately. A few weeks later, she can eat almost anything, whereas before she was limited to a handful of foods. It would be interesting to discover if the consumption of active yogurt cultures would reduce the effect of yeast mediated reactions. Certainly, active yogurt (as opposed to pasteurized yogurt) is effective in treatment of migraine, a yeast mediated disease.

Fiber is that component of food which cannot be digested. Fiber forms the bulk that helps us remain regular, but its importance is more than such a basic necessity. Fiber traps waste products discharged with bile into the small intestine, so that they can be removed from the body. The most infamous of these is toxic peroxidized cholesterol, which is made soluble by vitamin C and excreted via the liver in bile. Fiber also speeds the passage of waste products so that they do not have time to be resorbed into the body. This may be the major reason that high fiber diets are associated with a low incidence of cancer. There are several diseases associated with straining due to lack of bulk in the bowel, including hemorrhoids and diverticulosis, and fiber would prevent these.

Our diet probably contains the few essential fats, except in those persons who cannot absorb fats. Fat is essential, though, and every diet should have at least 9 grams of fat daily. Unless you are on a strict weight reduction diet, this is all too easy to attain. Essential fatty acids are altered by food processing to make them more stable, but unfortunately making them very toxic to cell membranes, the stuff of life itself. There are increasing reports of diseases caused by these essential fatty acid antagonists, which should not occur except in a diet rich in processed foods. The altered essential fatty acids are incorporated into the molecules of the cell membranes, producing a defective leaky membrane. In technical terms, the altered fatty acids result in a membrane that is permeable to ions it should block. The resulting influx of calcium and sodium into the cells, and loss of magnesium and potassium, is one cause of hypertension. If your cells are not functioning properly, you cannot function properly.

Vitamins are catalysts which our body cannot manufacture. They must therefore be eaten. Vitamins A and D are fat soluble, and can be stored in the body. Because they can be stored, it is possible to eat enough to produce toxic effects. The toxic levels are really quite high, and most persons cannot afford the expense of taking that much on a regular basis. Vitamin A can be produced in the body from carotenes, the yellow pigments which give carrots their color. Carotenes are water soluble, and therefore are not toxic. Other than the fact that they make the skin yellow they are perfectly safe. In fact, the beta carotenes are potent antioxidants and should be included in the daily diet. The body only converts enough to meet its vitamin A needs. Note, however, that diabetics generally cannot make this conversion to retinol, the fat soluble form of vitamin A. It is important to remember that vitamin A (retinol) does not replace the beta carotenes in their role as antioxidants. Both are required in the diet, whereas the beta carotenes are required daily while retinol can be stored for future needs. Although vitamin A can be stored in the liver, analysis of autopsy specimens in Canada has confirmed that 10 percent of those autopsied had no vitamin A stores. The USDA concluded in 1968 that 40 percent of Americans were deficient in vitamin A. A decade later, our diet has fewer sources of vitamin A than before.

Vitamin D is also stored and is toxic in excess. It is made in the body on exposure to sunlight. Synthetic vitamin D is added to so many foods that we all are getting far too much of this synthetic vitamin. Supplementation of vitamin D should always be with the natural form which has never produced toxic manifestations. I am now recommending that the natural vitamin D be taken whenever vitamin A is supplemented. The two seem to work together with better results. Supplementation with synthetic vitamin D in America is not recommended, but the natural form may be used safely in moderation.

There are numerous water soluble vitamins. These vitamins cannot be stored, and must be included in the daily diet. In some cases deficiency symptoms develop within a week of being deprived of water soluble vitamins. Most of these vitamins are lost if water used in preparation of foods is poured off. They are also generally sensitive to heat, and are lost upon cooking. These vitamins are a major reason why many vegetables should be eaten raw, and should never be overcooked. Steaming and cooking in a microwave oven are ideal ways to preserve the nutrition nature put in our foods.

We must come to realize that there is a vast difference between optimum health and just being alive. Long before clinical evidence of deficiencies develops, our bodies are no longer operating at peak efficiency. Like a car in need of fresh oil, the human body that has marginal nutrition has less pep and wears out sooner.

I hope that by now your mind is sufficiently open to examine your diet and take corrective action. After all, it is your life. This book will provide a useful roadmap as you explore optimum nutrition and reach towards optimum health. Good luck!

II.
The Education
of a Physician

Actually, this chapter is not about the gory details of medical education, nor the soap opera view of a doctor's life. This is about the education we all receive in the School of Life. I have learned through living that life is a classroom, and that the lessons given are useful and for a purpose. I have also learned that a lesson not learned is a lesson repeated. Once you realize what life is all about it becomes more interesting. The lessons I have to learn are not yours, nor or your lessons mine. However, it is a wise man who learns from another's lessons.

When I began my formal medical education two decades ago, the extent of nutritional education was: "The American diet contains all the necessary vitamins and minerals. Anyone taking additional vitamins is wasting his money." Medical education in nutrition has not improved since then. In fact, when I had occasion to visit my alma mater last year, I made it a point to visit the bookstore. There was not one book on nutrition. Of course, we had a good background in biochemistry, but no one seemed to apply this knowledge to what is happening in the patient who is trying to get well and stay well. The myth of the Perfect American Diet had blinded us all.

The first indication I had that the American diet was inadequate came when Clara and I dropped by through Waynesville to visit my former eighth-grade teacher, Mr. Roy Haupt. When I left Waynesville after graduating in 1959, Roy was in his mid-40s (I think), and looked at least ten years older. When we returned some four years later, he had trimmed up, his hair was darker, and he looked to be in his mid-30s. My exclamation on seeing him was, "Roy, what happened?!" It turns out that Roy had an eccentric neighbor, one of those health-food nuts. You know the kind. Finally, Roy had gotten tired of his constantly preaching nutrition to him and challenged him to make out a diet which Roy would follow for six months. If nothing happened, his friend was to shut up. Well, Roy said, "After about three months my waist began to get smaller, my hair began to thicken and darken, and I looked and felt years younger. If you think I am going to quit the diet now, you're crazy!"

This story also has a postscript. Recently I decided to drop by again and visit my old friend, Roy. He would now be in his late 60s, and I had not seen him for about twenty years. I expected to see an old man, perhaps senile, and didn't look forward to seeing my friend in that condition. Not to worry, as the Japanese say. Roy looked great. His mind was sharp as a tack, and he looked not a day over fifty. Roy does 150 pushups and 300 situps daily, and is enjoying life. This is much more than he could do when he was 45. Like a vintage wine, he has improved with age. Praise God. And pass the vitamins, please.

My education in nutrition continued in medical school, when I read in Christopher's *Textbook of Surgery* that patients whose wounds break open after surgery are almost always deficient in vitamin C. This book also stated that the requirements for vitamin C rose to as much as 10 grams a day under the stress of surgery or severe illness. Interestingly, most surgeons seem not to have read that simple fact, and have neglected to treat their patients with vitamin C before and after surgery. In over a decade of doing eye surgery, I have never had even one wound break open, although this complication is really very common. This truth has been proven time and again, and is still ignored by the majority of surgeons and physicians.

It only takes one day on intravenous glucose to totally deplete the body of thiamine and zinc, yet how rarely do physicians add vitamins to the intravenous solutions. And zinc, which is absolutely essential for healing is seldom given to those who need it most. A study recently done in Boston, and repeated in Atlanta, confirmed that the majority of patients admitted to the intensive care unit were malnourished, and were especially deficient in zinc. When the prognosis was compared, those with severe deficiencies generally died while those whose nutrition was better got well. Still few physicians use nutrition to prevent disease or speed recovery. Most are still blinded by the Utopian dream of American perfection.

During my obstetrics and gynecology rotation as an intern at the Portsmouth Naval Hospital in Virginia, I became aware of studies proving that 75 percent of spontaneous miscarriages were associated with folic acid deficiency. At the time, the pre-natal vitamin used by the Navy did not have folic acid in the formula. Lederle had just introduced Filabon FA, which had 400 micrograms of folic acid. The staff gave me the opportunity to present the evidence in favor of switching to Filabon FA, and as a result the entire U.S. Navy soon switched to using Filabon FA as the preferred prenatal vitamin. It would be interesting to know how many young men and women are alive today as a result of that wise decision by those physicians.

As well as I remember, the next clue that our diet is inadequate came during my tour of duty aboard a nuclear submarine. Commonly toward the end of patrols several of the crew would develop mouth ulcers and periodontal disease, resistant to antibiotics and mouth washes. It suddenly dawned on me that this looked a lot like the pictures of scurvy I had seen in my textbooks. Sure enough, every case cleared within forty-eight hours on vitamin C alone. On the second patrol with this crew, we had multi-vitamins on the table each breakfast, and only four men developed scurvy. None of the four had been taking the vitamins. By the third patrol the word had gotten around and no more cases occurred.

Scurvy in the nuclear Navy? Yes. And I am sure it is still there today, unless the word has finally gotten around throughout the fleet. What kind of man got scurvy at sea? It turns out that the only ones getting scurvy were bachelors who "lived on the beach." Beer, pretzels, and hamburgers are not a major source of vitamin C. They were borderline scorbutic on going to sea, and when within a few weeks our fresh vegetables were gone, their scurvy became manifest.

I did not think too much about nutrition again until my second year of residency in ophthalmology at the National Naval Medical Center in Bethesda, Maryland. One of my patients was a 68-year-old man who came in for a routine examination. Not that he felt any need for an eye exam, because he had better than 20/20 vision at distance and could also read at near as well as any teenager, *all* without glasses! I spent about an hour with him questioning him about his diet, his parents, everything. According to my textbooks, the ability to focus at near is always lost with age, yet here before me was a clear exception to the rule. It is the exceptions to the rule that teach us lessons, and I decided then that if one man could avoid aging, then so could another; and I might as well be that man. Later, while attending the Lanchester Course in ophthalmology at Colby College, I took the opportunity to ask one of the professors in refraction whether he had seen a similar situation where someone had avoided aging. In his thirty or so years of experience, yes, he had examined two or three such persons. What God had run by me was not an isolated experience.

During my residency, I was the only doctor in our program who used vitamins before and after surgery. One of the staff members was particularly upset that I did such a thing, and hounded me constantly. Nevertheless, it was also recognized that I had better surgical results than most of the other surgeons. One day during a bull session, he challenged me openly before the group. My answer ended the harrassment: "We all recognize that I have fewer complications and better results than anyone else here. Now it is either the result of the vitamins or I am a better surgeon than you are. You pick which one you think it is." Silence.

During this time we seemed to have a lot of cases of central serous macular edema, perhaps because it is related to stress, and we were, after all, in the Washington area. Stress abounds there. There was no effective treatment of the disease at that time, although today the laser can be used effectively in selected cases. Generally, it is a self-limiting disease, though many never fully recover their vision. I discovered that many of the persistent cases could be treated with vitamin C plus bioflavinoids, both of which are necessary to protect the integrity of small vessel walls, the problem area in this disease. With this treatment many had their vision return to them in spite of being unable to see for years. Of course, there were many failures. But that does not detract from the successes.

During this time, my wife's sister also lived in the Washington area, and we visited her after several months without getting together. She was obviously younger in appearance, and radiated health. Not being totally stupid in my old age, I started the questions. It turned out that she had begun taking vitamin E about two months before, and had noticed that after about six weeks she no longer awakened exhausted, and that she slept about two hours less than before. The change in her appearance was remarkable, so Clara and I began taking vitamin E. We, too, noted that after about six weeks we were requiring less sleep, and were more active. I was at that time with the Armed Forces Institute of Pathology, and had begun swimming during my lunch hour. This was after we had already noticed the benefits. Remarkably, even though I pushed myself to the limits of endurance, my muscles did not get sore. I passed this information along to another physician, who began on 1000 IU of vitamin E daily, and pushed himself as hard as possible. He was swimming a mile during the lunch hour within a week, and also had no soreness. Since then, I have effectively used vitamin E before and after strenuous work to prevent muscle soreness, with almost universal success. It is more effective taken before the fact, but is also effective after the stress. It should come as no surprise that all of the Olympic champions in recent years have taken vitamin E during training and competition.

I became aware of the importance of trace elements during this period. I have a cousin who raises beef and dairy cattle, and during one visit he told me that cattle raised on pasture-land that is intensively fertilized over several years will die. Intensive fertilization over a period of years depletes the soil of trace minerals, and the grass grows green, but can no longer sustain animal life. The solution is to add ocean salt to the diet of the cattle. Since the ocean is the reservoir of eons of soil erosion, salt from the ocean would contain all the minerals previously present in the soil. It did not take me long to realize that all the vegetables now on the market are raised on intensively farmed soil just as that grass is. We are not that different from cattle, and should be suffering with the same problems. We are not because we are getting our minerals from eating the cattle.

Our family immediately switched to using sea salt instead of mined salt. Six months later, I began to notice that my ability to focus at near was returning. When I was 32, I had six diopters of accommodation, about average for that age. It had increased to 10 diopters, typical of someone under twenty. It is still over eight diopters, typical of someone in their early 20s, and I am 44 years old. When I am rested I can still crank in 10 diopters of power.

Incidently, there are several excellent sources of these trace elements. Sea salt is perhaps best. The idea is not to heavily salt everything in sight, but to put sea salt in your shaker, and use it just as you would any ordinary salt. Unfortunately, what is passed off as sea salt at many health food stores is evaporated salt which has had the valuable trace elements removed for separate sale. True sea salt is rather coarse and has an off color. Unadulterated sea salt is rich in magnesium, and has very little aluminum or iron. An analysis will determine whether the salt you have purchased is genuine sea salt or has had its valuable minerals extracted. Mineral salt from a farm supply store may or may not be equivalent to true sea salt. Some of it is mined with added trace elements, and will show high levels of iron and aluminum on analysis. If analysis shows it to be good, it can be made acceptable for table use by grinding it in a blender or salt grinder.

Alfalfa grows with its roots running over forty feet into the earth, and brings up trace minerals at depth, minerals that are not available in the intensively farmed surface soil. This may be why even a small amount of alfalfa sprinkled in a garden will dramatically improve production. Not only does alfalfa contain trace minerals, but it is a valuable source of dietary fiber, with all its benefits. It is the best source of silicon which may be the key deficiency in degenerative diseases. I would recommend taking at least six alfalfa tablets daily in addition to using mineral salt. Less expensive, perhaps more effective, and certainly more tasty would be to sprout alfalfa sprouts at home and use them as a filler for meat dishes and salads.

Another way of getting trace elements is to add it to your garden by using green sand, an ocean mineral rich in potassium and trace elements in a form that is slowly released. Seaweed can also be used. Body Toddy™ is a superior commercial product.

Sea foods are a third source of trace elements other than the obvious one of direct supplements. All ocean life is rich in trace elements, and those higher up the food chain are richer sources. This does not apply to fresh water fish. Seafoods are expensive, but should be included in your diet regularly.

In 1974, I had the good fortune to be assigned to Ethiopia with the International Eye Foundation to help set up a facility for eye surgery. This was a valuable experience, not only surgically and culturally, but concerning nutrition. It seemed that Ethiopia was a land of blind people. Almost everyone over forty had cataracts, glaucoma was common, and even the children had eye diseases common to those with vitamin A deficiencies. I became convinced that the early onset of cataracts there was the result of diet, and that if it were diet there, it probably was due to diet in the U.S. I began then trying various dietary approaches to reversing cataracts, none of which worked.

I had finally given up on finding a solution when in 1978 a patient came to me with bilateral 20/200 cataracts. He was blind in each eye. I scheduled surgery and successfully removed one cataract, but because he was a bachelor, and remembering my Navy experience about bachelors, I put him on a new vitamin product identical to a vitamin product I had used previously, except that it had zinc added to it. I used the supplements in hopes that he would heal faster so that I could operate on his other eye. Instead, the vision in the other eye improved to 20/25 over a six-month period of time. He still has 20/25 vision in that eye four years later.

It so happened that on the day he returned with his excellent vision, another lady also had made an appointment for treatment of her cataracts. She had 20/60 vision in each eye: ready for surgery. Instead, I put her on the vitamins plus zinc and waited six weeks. She returned with 20/30 vision. She no longer needed surgery, so we waited another six weeks. This time she could see 20/20 in each eye! I immediately stopped all cataract surgery until my patients could have the opportunity to benefit from this discovery.

The last time I checked my records, 67 percent of those treated had improved vision, and over 50 percent of those who initially needed cataract surgery, improved to the point where surgery was no longer needed. This was with nothing more than a simple vitamin/mineral supplement containing zinc. So another lesson in life was learned: obviously our diet is not so perfect as I had been taught in medical school.

Soon after we returned to Western North Carolina, my younger son, George, had a bicycle accident and suffered a considerable loss of skin from both elbows. This did not heal for three years, so that even a minor injury to his elbows would cause it to bleed and be very painful. Twice I excised the scar tissue and closed the wound; but George is an active boy, and the scar was soon broken open again. I realized that the only way to cure the problem was to again excise it and this time put his arm in a cast until it had healed. Instead, I recalled the use of vitamin E for burn patients to speed healing and to soften scars. So I put him on 400 IU of vitamin E three times daily. Within three days the wound had healed and has given him no trouble in the years since. Our family had not been taking vitamin E since about 1975, but we immediately began again and have not stopped since.

Later, I had the good fortune to read a book about vitamin E written by Dr. Shute. I cannot rewrite his book here, and will not attempt to do so. I can, however, tell how this has affected my practice of ophthalmology. One of the things Dr. Shute claims for vitamin E is its ability to stop inflamation, such as in phlebitis. In ophthalmology, one of the common complications after cataract surgery is cystoid macular edema, which is thought to be the result of inflammation. So I started giving my patients 400 IU of vitamin E immediately after surgery, and noticed that they recovered much faster than before. Next, I increased the dosage to 400 IU three times daily, and began treatment the day before surgery. Immediately, I began to have patients whose vision recovered within a few days of surgery rather than after many weeks. At present, I use the product Basic Preventive (TM) made by AMNI, plus an additional 1200 IU of vitamin E. According to Dr. Cranton, the addition of glutathione should improve my results still further. This will be the next step in my attempt to reduce inflammation after eye surgery.

I have one patient who had had cataract surgery by another physician several years ago, whose initial good results deteriorated to dismal within a few weeks. When I initially saw her, her vision in that eye had been mere count fingers for years. I sent her to a retina specialist, who confirmed that she was permanently and incurably blind in that eye. On vitamin/mineral therapy, her vision began to improve within five months, and by nine months she could see well enough to pass a driver's examination. She now has 20/25 vision in that eye.

Another patient was one who had reacted to eye surgery with intense inflammation, which I had been unable to control even with intensive steroid therapy over a period of several weeks. I put him on 1600 IU of vitamin E daily, and within three days the eye was quiet and comfortable.

Lessons continue to come. In 1982, I had switched to a sustained release vitamin/mineral product that had a very high level of vitamin A. Some of my cataract patients also had glaucoma, and I had noticed that some of these patients were enjoying a marked reduction of pressure in their eyes. In December, 1982, an article appeared in a glaucoma journal demonstrating vitamin A deficiency in glaucoma patients, confirming my serendipitous findings.

One patient had a dermatological disease which was a real curse. He looked like he had been bathed in glue and sprinkled with corn flakes. He had been treated for years by a dermatologist, but to no avail. I had put him on vitamins and zinc for his eye problems, and within a few months his skin disease began to abate. It never completely cleared, but it did clear so substantially that he was able to discontinue all other medications. His problem was mainly nutritional.

It does not take too many such cases to convince an open minded person that our nutrition is inadequate. I will therefore give one more personal story, then close this introduction.

In early December, 1982, I had occasion to check my personal calcium intake, and discovered that I was getting only 50 percent of the RDA of calcium. I looked up the symptoms of calcium deficiency, and found that I had several, including hypertension and chronic back pain (due to osteoporosis). My hypertension had been a matter of concern for over five years, since three physicians had been unable to bring it under control without circulatory collapse—which had occurred three times during this period, and had nearly caused my death at least twice. I had finally settled out with a blood pressure of 145/110, since that was as low as we could get it safely.

I started looking around for a palatable source of calcium, and discovered a soybean protein supplement which was rich in calcium. Add a few calcium/magnesium tablets to that, and I have met my RDA for calcium and gotten a good breakfast in the process. Enthused, our whole family began on the new diet for breakfast.

We immediately noticed several positive effects: first, my wife and I were no longer starved out of our everloving minds by lunchtime, and I began to lose weight. A definite plus. Second, my two sons had been coming home after school tired and hard to live with. In fact, they frequently had to be separated until supper in order to maintain peace. The hostility and irritability simply disappeared. We ran out of the protein supplement during the Christmas holidays, and could hardly wait until we could get a fresh supply. If for no other reason, the peace in the family brought on by good nutrition has been worth every penny. Good nutrition does not cost, it pays!

Later, long term benefits began to appear. Our fingernails have become harder, and our hair is growing faster. Now I have to have a haircut weekly rather than once a month as heretofore. My barber likes that. My weight has continued to drop, and now I have lost about twenty pounds since I can take advantage of the fact that the protein breakfast has eliminated hunger pangs. My waist is five inches smaller, and although I weigh ten pounds more than I did when I had my suits tailored in 1977, I fit these suits perfectly today. Not only have I lost fat, but I have obviously gained muscle. After about two months, I noted that my blood pressure was also dropping, and it has now dropped to 110/70, which is perfectly normal. A few weeks ago a study was released in the *Journal of the American Medical Association* showing that calcium supplementation results in a drop in blood pressure in hypertensive persons after about six weeks of therapy with one gram of calcium daily. Other studies have shown that supplementation with two grams of calcium daily results in a dramatic drop in blood cholesterol. (Supplementation with over 2 grams daily is not advised.) It should be pointed out here that our requirement for extra calcium is largely due to our distorted diet, which drains us of dietary calcium and also causes inappropriate (and harmful) calcium deposits. Long term high calcium consumption will block the uptake of essential trace elements, and thus produce other deficiencies.

So finally, I am thoroughly convinced that the Perfect American Diet is mere fiction. I do not think it is possible, much less likely, that anyone can consume adequate amounts of vitamins and minerals in an unsupplemented diet. I have tried, and have been unable to produce a diet that would meet even the RDA, much less the larger amounts of most vitamins that I am convinced we need to remain healthy.

The remainder of this book will be dedicated to giving my present opinions about what is adequate nutrition. I admit from the onset that I will not be able to present proof of my statements. All I can say is that reason, unblinded by prejudice, has made it amply clear that we are a nation of malnourished people. Our hospitals and nursing homes are full of the results of our folly. Widespread deficiencies exist for most of the vitamins and especially the elements calcium, chromium, magnesium, manganese, selenium, silicon, vanadium, and zinc. This is a time of intensive research into the benefits of nutrition. Much will be learned in the next few years. The benefits will be the end of degenerative diseases, optimum health, and a greatly expanded lifespan. A healthy, active life of 120 years is not unlikely. This is the limit on man placed by God several thousand years ago (Genesis 6:3), and is the same limit recently discovered by scientists investigating aging. It is a reasonable goal, already proven by nutrition experiments with animals.

I do believe that this is God's will, and that this generation will live to see it fulfilled. This book is but one small step in that direction. Enjoy the life God has given you to the fullest. That is his will for you.

III.
Free Radical Pathology

Every few generations an insight so profound comes along that it cuts through the veil clouding our minds and puts into perspective a confusing collection of observations and facts. Mendel's discovery of the basic rules of genetics was one such insight. So was the discovery of bacteria and their role in infection.

Free radical pathology, first put forth by Dr. Denham Harman three decades ago, is such a discovery which promises to tie together a lot of loose ends in degenerative diseases: everything from arthritis and atherosclerosis, to diabetes and aging.

Free radicals, as used here, is not a term describing members of the Weather Underground who have not been apprehended. A free radical, in its simplest term, is an atom or molecule which has an unpaired electron in its outer shell, and is therefore highly reactive. A free radical is an accident looking for a place to happen, so to speak. Free radicals are both essential for life processes, and highly destructive to life. Controlled within the mitochondria (organelles within each cell), free radicals release energy for useful work. Free radicals are also a necessary result of detoxifying many chemicals, including drugs, petrochemicals (in smog, for example), artificial flavors and colorings, and rancid fats. In fact, your leucocytes (white cells) use free radicals to kill invading bacteria. Outside this controlled environment, free radicals destroy cellular membranes, genetic material, enzymes, and life itself. We are not unaccustomed to such a concept, for the fire contained within a furnace warms the home and soul, but uncontrolled the same fire can turn that home into a smoldering pile of ashes. Virtually everything useful is potentially dangerous, even lethal. That is the nature of life. Controlling these forces is what life is all about both at the molecular and cellular level, as well as at the level of society and the individual.

Since most of the free radicals to which we are exposed are transported via blood, it is only natural that the walls of blood vessels suffer most from their attack. An atheroma, the beginning stage of degenerative blood vessel disease, is essentially a benign tumor growing in the wall of a blood vessel. As it enlarges, it outgrows its blood supply (it must get its nutrients directly from the blood), and necroses (dies) within. This dead tissue within the atheroma accumulates calcium deposits which further hardens the walls of the blood vessel. The atheroma causes damage by restricting blood flow (which produces anoxia, which produces more free radicals), and by becoming a nidus for the formation of a thrombosis (blood clot) which we have already seen to be activated by free radicals. Once free radical activity is controlled, natural healing processes will diminish the size of any atheroma present.

Malignancy is caused when free radicals react with cellular DNA and alter the genetic material of a cell. If the damage is located at a critical place, the cell multiplies out of control, possibly producing death.

If the free radical damage is to a less critical part of DNA, or to RNA, abnormal enzymes or proteins are produced and cell function is compromised. If the attack is on a cell membrane, the membrane ceases to function and becomes leaky, allowing essential ions to leak out of the cell, or ions which should remain outside the cell to leak in. Loss of cellular chromium in this manner is one cause of adult onset diabetes. The ensuing loss of cellular potassium and magnesium and the influx of sodium and calcium are a major cause of hypertension. (Essential fatty acids which have been altered by food processors also result in leaky cell membranes. Evening primrose oil is one source of unaltered essential fatty acids.)

Free radical damage to collagen causes the cross-linkage of collagen molecules, and the loss of elasticity. Wrinkled skin, stiff joints, and hypertension are natural results. Silicon in the diet seems to protect collagen against cross-linkage.

In the mitochondria (which are organelles within each cell) free radicals are neutralized by an enzyme named superoxide dismutase (SOD). This enzyme contains manganese, which is frequently deficient in the American diet. Outside the mitochondria, another form of SOD is used which contains both zinc and copper. Another scavenging enzyme, glutathione peroxidase requires four atoms of selenium. Both selenium and zinc are common deficiencies. Free radicals are also produced within the body through reactions in which iron or copper act as catalysts. Since both copper and iron are parts of different enzymes which function to scavenge free radicals, they are essential to life. But in excess, both produce free radicals. This property of iron and copper to be both friend and foe makes it urgent that they should never be supplemented without first demonstrating a deficiency by laboratory test.

In addition to the enzymes mentioned above, certain vitamins and elements function as free radical scavengers. Vitamin E's only function may be to intercept free radicals and reduce them to a non-toxic form. In the process, vitamin E is oxidized to tocoperol quinone. Oxidized vitamin E is recycled to tocoperol by vitamin C, which, in turn, is oxidized to dehydroascorbate. Dehydroascorbate is recycled to vitamin C by the enzyme glutathione peroxidase (which requires selenium). Glutathione peroxidase is restored to its active form by oxidizing reduced glutathione, which, in turn, is reduced again by a riboflavin-dependent enzyme, glutathione reductase. This enzyme is reactivated by NADH, a niacin containing enzyme. The result is oxidized NAD, which enters normal metabolic pathways and produces useful energy or work.

It is important to note that the detoxification of a free radical requires several elements and vitamins, all present and working together. Obviously, if the diet is deficient in one element or enzyme in this complex chain of reactions, supplementing with one of the other elements will produce minimal benefits. This is why attempts to determine the benefit of isolated nutrients have frequently produced equivocal results. It is as irrational as trying to determine the effect of food while simultaneously depriving the subject of oxygen. The ensuing death may have very little to do with a lack of calories.

Dietary items which are effective free radical scavengers include beta carotene, vitamin E, vitamin C, selenium (which is effective as an element and in its associated enzyme), cysteine (which is used in the synthesis of glutathione), riboflavin, and niacin. One of the most dangerous free radical forms is singlet oxygen (not paired as the usual oxygen molecule), for which we have no internal defense systems. Singlet oxygen is the result of overloaded internal defense systems (SOD), or exposure to pollutants such as tobacco smoke. The most effective and perhaps only substance for neutralizing the oxygen free radical is beta carotene, which effectively explains why dietary beta carotenes are associated with a markedly reduced cancer risk. It is important to note that although beta carotene is a precursor of vitamin A, vitamin A does *not* have this protective ability.

Radiation, a major fear among many today, injures and kills through the production of free radicals. The free radicals produced by radiation *are not different* than those produced by rancid foods, pollution, or normal metabolism. In fact, free radicals in our diet and internally produced are a much greater risk than would have occurred by living inside the Three Mile Island nuclear plant at the time of the radiation leak. Free radical pathology is so rampant that aging and degenerative diseases could be considered the end result of an internal nuclear meltdown.

How do free radicals produce such diverse pathologies? In the case of cancer, free radicals reacting with DNA produce an abnormal replication of genetic material, which may result in a malignant transformation. In reacting with lubricants within the joints, or with collagen within tendons and ligaments, there is a reduction in lubrication within the joint, or in elasticity on the connecting tissues. The results include joint pains and arthritis. The combination of all these activities of free radicals results in what is commonly called the aging process. If the tissues in the walls of blood vessels are involved, then atherosclerosis is the unavoidable result.

In one situation, peroxidized fats (a fatty free radical) are proven to inhibit an enzyme (prostacyclin) which prevents blood from clotting within a blood vessel. Peroxidized fats, which become concentrated in diseased arterial walls (made that way by free radical damage), increase the probability that a blood clot will form at the diseased site. In the process of clot formation, blood cells rupture and release both iron and copper, which act as catalysts to further peroxidation of fats, which goes through the cycle and causes the clot to extend. This explains why a meal rich in peroxidized fats can trigger a myocardial infarction (heart attack), and why heavy supplementation with vitamin E (which helps prevent the formation of peroxidized fats) will reduce the risk of such attacks (myocardial infarctions, strokes, and venous thrombosis).

There is a simple test to determine the amount of damage you have sustained from free radicals. Extend your hand, without tightening the skin. Grasp the skin on the back of your hand with your other hand, and lift the fold upwards. Release the fold of skin and notice how fast it snaps back into position. In a young person, or anyone with minimal free radical damage, the skin will snap back immediately. When there is considerable damage due to cross linkage of collagen (a connective tissue found throughout the body), the skin fold will slowly slip back into place, sometimes taking several seconds. Try this test on yourself, on a young person's skin, and on an elderly person. The degeneration demonstrated by this test is occurring throughout the body, and is reversible by proper nutrition and perhaps additionally chelation therapy.

Several years ago, it was noted that persons who have a crease in the skin of the ear lobe are more prone to heart disease. This crease is the result of free radical cross-linkage of collagen molecules.

A third test for free radical damage must be ordered by your physician. Cholesterol is one of the body's defenses against free radicals, and is produced internally in response to free radical levels. Reduced (beneficial) cholesterol is bound to a high density lipoprotein molecule (HDL). When it reacts with a free radical, the peroxidized cholesterol molecule becomes toxic, and is bound to a low density lipoprotein molecule (LDL). This toxic cholesterol is removed by the liver and excreted in bile. Vitamin C is essential for its elimination. Dietary fiber is essential to prevent the excreted toxic cholesterol from being resorbed. By testing for total cholesterol and for LDL and HDL cholesterol, the physician can determine your free radical status. Ideally, the LDL should be low, and the majority of your cholesterol should be the reduced type which is bound to HDL. Any level of total cholesterol greater than 150 probably indicates free radical activity, but only levels above about 200 are statistically associated with an increased risk of heart disease.

Where are all these free radicals coming from? Certainly, it is not a Communist plot to destroy us all. It is perhaps more a matter of internal subversion and fifth column activities. As indicated above, free radicals are a part of normal metabolism, and are controlled within the mitochondria if proper nutrients are available. Without these free radicals we would die, so we will not concern ourselves about them as a separate source.

The major sources of free radicals include natural and manmade radiation (X-rays, gamma rays, and the like), peroxidized dietary fats (*all* unsaturated and rancid fats), ozone, internal oxidation of fats, alcohol (which is metabolized to acetaldehyde, which generates free radicals), aromatic hydrocarbons within tobacco smoke, chlorinated water, and cadmium within drinking water and tobacco smoke. Already mentioned are dietary excesses of iron and copper, which, like cadmium, are free radical catalysts. Anoxia (too little oxygen) produces free radicals. Anoxia, of course, can occur with injury or reduced cardiac/lung function, and always occurs when we get insufficient exercise. Hyperbaric oxygen suppresses the free radical process, both

24

directly and by reducing anoxia. Also, hyperbaric oxygen increases the activity of superoxide dismutase (SOD), which in turn helps control free radical activity. In addition, all free radicals catalyse the production of additional free radicals, and can increase their concentration a million-fold in seconds. Incidently, peroxidized cholesterol is an extremely toxic free radical, and is bound preferentially to low density lipoproteins (LDL). Reduced cholesterol is a potent scavenger of free radicals (at which time it becomes peroxidized), and is preferentially bound to high density lipoproteins (HDL). An egg yolk in which the yolk membrane is intact is an excellent source of beneficial reduced cholesterol. If the yolk is broken in the cooking process, the cholesterol is oxidized and becomes very toxic. Thus an egg boiled, poached, or sunny side up is wholesome; whereas, it is toxic when scrambled or used in an omelet, or cooked in cakes or custards.

Of the sources mentioned above, peroxidized fats are by far the most common and dangerous source. Fats become peroxidized (transformed into free radicals) upon exposure to oxygen (in the air), during metabolism, and especially upon exposure to air while being heated. Fat stored within the body also oxidizes into toxic lipid peroxides, so fat is dangerous when it is eaten and when it is stored as excess weight. Metal ions, especially iron and copper, speed the process. Not only does this combination of factors peroxidize fats, but it also produces an isomerization of the fat molecule which then gets incorporated into cell membranes producing a defective membrane. But that is another problem, not directly related to free radical damage.

Unsaturated fats, those vegetable oils so highly touted and advertised, are most easily oxidized. To manufacture these oils without toxic peroxidation would require cold pressing in an inert atmosphere devoid of oxygen, and in the presence of additional vitamin E. It is possible, but not economically feasible. The worst of all worlds is the reuse of cooking oils, especially for frying, and especially where the oil is kept hot for hours on end. This is exactly the situation where fried foods are cooked in fast food restaurants. Obviously, you will use unsaturated oils in preparation of foods. Buy them in small glass containers, use them promptly, and never reuse them. Antioxidants such as BHT could be added to oils to reduce this toxic reaction.

Saturated fats, those found in animal fats and butter, are less easily peroxidized, but will oxidize if the temperatures are high enough. The flavor of grilled meat is due to saturated fats which become peroxidized upon contact with hot burning charcoal.

Nevertheless, saturated fats are safer than unsaturated fats, especially if used in moderation. Butter, a natural saturated fat, is much safer than margarine which not only contains high levels of peroxidized fats, but contains those modified fat molecules which produce leaky cellular membranes. So much for good intentions.

Vitamin C appears to be the major defense against free radical damage within the brain, eye, and central nervous system. It is so important, in fact, that there is a natural pump mechanism which increases the concentration of vitamin C in those tissues to many times that in other parts of the body. Anoxia, as caused by stroke, injury, or heart attack, produces a rapid increase of free radicals within the brain to lethal levels. Vitamin C, if present before the injury, will reduce the extent of injury. DMSO, an extremely potent synthetic free radical scavenger also protects tissue during injury. Hydergine (Sandoz) likewise has been proven to delay central nervous system damage during anoxia. Routine administration of vitamin C and Hydergine during labor and delivery would probably have very beneficial effects on the health of the child. (Vitamin E does not pass the placental barrier and would not be immediately beneficial, except to the mother.)

Is there any evidence that antioxidant compounds prolong life and reduce aging (and other free radical pathology)? Yes, there is. Mice fed food preserved with antioxidants live longer. More importantly, the effect extended to offspring when the antioxidants were used before mating. Santoquin,™ a feed antioxidant made by Monsanto for the poultry industry, displays some interesting effects which may prove the point of argument being made. Unfortunately, definitive answers will take years to establish.

A practical defense strategy against free radical pathology will be discussed in a later chapter. In the meantime, buy your French fries from McDonald's, the only company with the courage to stay with the best in spite of bad (and unfair) press. McDonald's uses saturated fats for frying, the safest way to go if you must fry.

IV.
Fiber

I have chosen fiber as one of my first topics for discussion because it is the most likely to be ignored, and very well may be the most important factor in overall health. The role of fiber is actually an area of considerable controversy in the medical community. In spite of the controversy, through, many facts are clear.

Fiber is most recognized as necessary for regular bowel function. Needless to say, a diet of highly processed foods will be almost totally digestible, and will leave virtually nothing to pass on through the bowels. Nor will fiber alone move things along: fiber is but one of the factors designed into our system by our Creator. You should not expect to function well without fiber any more than an automobile can function without oil. Exercise and water are essential for fiber to have its maximum benefit; all three must go together in a partnership for good health. It should also be pointed out that fiber is not fiber, so to speak. That is, natural fiber not only provides bulk necessary for bowel regularity, but valuable trace elements such as chromium, zinc, and silicon. There are breads on the market today which have added cellulose (from wood pulp) to improve the fiber content of the bread. Whereas this will serve to provide bulk, it will not provide the trace elements present in natural fiber products. If you are planning to supplement your diet with a fiber product, read the label carefully to discover the origin of the fiber. If possible, choose a product with fiber from various sources, such as pectin and bran.

Let's take it from the top. In the mouth, fiber helps scrub plaque off the teeth and keep the gums healthy. In the small intestine, fiber traps cholesterol and water in the intestine so that the bulk remains soft. In the process, much cholesterol is removed from the body. There may be other toxic products removed in the same manner.

Bacteria normally present in the large intestine act on the contents of the bowel and produce many by-products. Some, such as vitamin K, are essential to life. Unfortunately, toxic and carcinogenic substances are also produced in significant quantities whenever bowel action is sluggish. For example, toxic peroxidized cholesterol is excreted in the bile (with the aid of vitamin C), and is normally trapped in dietary fiber and excreted. If the diet is deficient in fiber, this highly toxic form of cholesterol is resorbed into the body.

The average American diet is highly refined, and contains less than three grams of fiber per day. The daily diet of primitive peoples generally has over 10 grams of fiber. Whether or not this is the reason, there are several diseases to which we Americans fall prey, which do not exist in areas where the diet contains ample fiber. These include appendicitis, diverticulosis and diverticulitis, hemorrhoids, atherosclerosis, cancer of the colon, and breast cancer. Why breast cancer? It has been shown that breast cancer is forty times more likely to occur in women who are constipated, or are not regular. The cancer seems to be due to carcinogenic substances produced in the colon, absorbed into the blood, and apparently concentrated in the breast. It may be due to silicon deficiencies which occur in a diet lacking fiber, or to vitamin E which is more plentiful in the primitive diet. Again, resorbed toxic cholesterol may be the villain.

Two of the most common cancers afflicting modern man would virtually disappear with the simple addition of fiber to the diet: these are cancer of the colon, and cancer of the breast.

We probably wouldn't get to enjoy all those "Preparation H™" television ads if everyone included sufficient fiber in their diet. And since a major source of bad breath is malodorous chemicals, mainly peroxidized (rancid) fatty acids, absorbed from the intestine and released through the lungs, we would also miss the battles between Scope™ and Listerine.™

The Israelis have shown that the toxins produced in the large intestine by the Candida albicans yeast can cause migraine headaches in susceptible persons. This can be corrected by overwhelming the undesirable bacteria with "good" bacteria by eating fresh yogurt, or by adding fiber to the diet to shorten the passage time. I recommend both to my patients with migraine, with good effect. Obviously, avoiding those conditions which promote yeast overgrowth (refined carbohydrates, antibiotics) and treatment of the Candida infection would also be beneficial.

Mechanically, a high fiber diet can reduce the likelihood of hemorrhoids, appendicitis, diverticulosis, and constipation. In the process, it will also reduce blood levels of the LDL toxic peroxidized cholesterol (the bad kind) and make atherosclerosis and gallstones less likely. Additionally, by eliminating constipation the risk of cancer of the colon and breast are greatly reduced. For those who suffer from migraine, about four out of five will find relief with nothing more than the fiber in an apple a day.

What are the sources of fiber? Almost anything you grow in your own garden and prepare for the table will provide fiber. Fresh fruit is especially good. Apples are rich in pectin, a type of fiber that traps water especially well. Bran cereals are made with the part of the grain that should never have been removed in the first place. Bran is the outer husk of the grain, and not only contains fiber, but many vitamins and minerals.

To be effective, fiber should be included in every meal. A meal rich in vegetables fresh from the garden probably has sufficient fiber. A breakfast of pancakes (made with highly refined flour) and eggs will have little fiber. Neither will the average lunch at a fast food restaurant. If your supper is steak and potatoes, then expect to feel sluggish the next day, poisoned by your own colon. Indeed, Grandma's castor oil treatment was not such a bad idea. I've had both, and will take an herbal laxative any time over castor oil, and fiber over either!

For those on a diet, fiber supplements will satisfy the need to chew while preventing the bane of most diets: constipation.

Incidently, you should learn to listen to your body: it is trying to tell you something. When you eat highly refined foods, or get the majority of your calories from animal proteins, you will become sluggish mentally and physically. I call it a satiated feeling. It is similar to the way you feel after feasting on Thanksgiving Day. Many persons have never felt any other way, and will not recognize what I am describing: the last thing a fish would discover would be water.

That is not the important thing. The satiated sensation is not a healthy one, and it needs to be recognized and corrected. It is corrected by increasing dietary fiber and water, severely curtailing calories (dieting or fasting for one or two days), and even taking a mild, but effective, herbal laxative. However, let me warn you that to fast or go on a restricted diet without first purging your system is to invite some of the problems brought on by colonic stasis. Enter your diet by increasing your fiber and water intake and using a laxative for one or two days. I do not recommend daily use of any laxative, although I am satisfied that herbal laxatives produce a natural movement, without discomfort or urgency. Vitamin C, pantothenic acid, and magnesium (which works with pyridoxine) also stimulate healthy bowel function. In this manner, left over animal proteins do not just sit there while your diet provides nothing to move things along.

In conclusion, fiber has been ignored too long. You should begin on it while you are young to prevent degenerative diseases older citizens wish they could have avoided. You will appreciate the advantages more when you are older and simple things become a pleasure. Your body was designed to have fiber, and fiber is necessary for good health. Neglect it at your own peril!

V.
Weight Control

It is estimated that at least 30 percent of the American population is overweight, and most of these have either tried dieting to lose weight, or are thinking about it. If you are not one of these, you almost certainly will be at some future date, because every food processor in the country is trying to get you to eat his product, and is using every psychological trick known to man to induce you to eat more. As a result, weight control is a common subject of advertising and featured articles in magazines, as we should expect of anything touching 30 percent of the population.

In simplest terms, being overweight is a matter of too many calories eaten, and too few burned. However, weight control is not as simple as that, for some people are very efficient in using calories, and require less food. Even worse, the body is very efficient in regulating energy consumption, and when put on a starvation diet switches to more efficient metabolic pathways to keep from losing fat. Thus the dieter who pulls weight off too quickly finds that he now gains weight on fewer calories than before. This disturbing discovery is very recent, and its ramifications are not yet known. It would appear, however, that the prudent dieter will opt for long term slow weight loss rather than try to pull the fat off by severely restrictive diets. Further, since weight control is really a task of behavior modification, a severe diet will not fit the bill. Short relative fasts of 700 or so highly nutritious calories daily will reset the appetite while not triggering the efficiency mechanism. My guess is that it takes at least a week to trigger this mechanism, and perhaps as long as six weeks. In years past, I have restricted my diet severely for as long as eight weeks without rebound weight gain, but more recently I restricted my caloric intake for several months and found that I was not losing weight even on fewer than a thousand calories daily. When I returned to about 1800 calories per day, I quickly regained what I had lost. Previously, this weight was maintained with about 3300 calories daily. You shouldn't try to fool Mother Nature.

As a result of this error, I regrouped and began looking for a better way to approach weight control. This has led to several insights which appear to be successful. First, I had to understand why I ate, just as you need to analyse why you are eating. "Of course," you would say, "I eat because I am hungry." Probably not. How often do you pick at your meal, or complain that you want something else rather than what is before you? That desire is more the result of an addiction, than true hunger. If you are truly hungry, you will probably eat anything set before you, and go out scrounging for more. What passes for hunger in most of us is no more than habit, the Pavlovian result of eating whenever the table is set. Advertising is based upon the principle that desire can be triggered by presenting the proper stimulus in an appealing manner. How often have you wanted a beer after a beer commercial on TV, even though you do not drink? A table set with a meal will trigger saliva and hunger pangs just as efficiently as a TV commercial, even if you are not hungry. So consider habit as your enemy. If you are not hungry, don't expose yourself to stimuli which will make you want to eat. Do something constructive instead: take a walk, jog, go to the Y and swim, read a book, or catch up on back work. Do anything, but stay out of the kitchen!

So we see that whereas hunger is triggered by the need for food, appetite is triggered by mainly psychological factors. In fact, you can be truly hungry and have no appetite, as you will shortly see. Appetite causes us to want to eat, and is triggered by several factors, including hunger in its early stages. However, appetite is also triggered by overeating, so it is not a dependable guide to eating. Psychological factors which trigger appetite include habit, the sight or smell of food, discussing food, or even merely thinking about food. I can also assure you that writing about food such as I am now creates an almost insatiable desire to eat. A little planning can help you turn these factors into friends. Since the stimulus which usually tricks us into eating when we are not hungry is habit (it is time to eat), then plan other activities during that period. Ask yourself *each time* before eating, "Am I hungry?" If you are not, then don't eat, and don't subject yourself to stimuli which will trigger your appetite. If you make dieting a test of will power you will surely lose, as you have surely lost up until this point.

Another factor forcing us to eat is sociological, and it very well may be the most difficult to avoid. For example, what reasonable recourse does a man have when his wife has slaved hours in a hot kitchen preparing a delicious meal and presenting it attractively? To say he is not hungry at such a time is to greatly strain the bonds of matrimony! The same applies when you are invited out to dinner with friends or business associates. Generations of scarcity of food has produced traditions and customs built around food. Business deals are most often closed over meals, and diplomacy is smoothed by banquets. With such a rich tradition we have a difficult battle indeed! It has only been in very recent years that food has become plentiful, at least in America. Somehow, we must learn to adjust to the new reality of plentiful food. How many times were you told as a child to clean your plate because there were children in China who were starving? Even the children of our poorest families have this common experience. One solution is to waste it, rather than waist it. A dog helps. A better solution is to prepare less, and to put less on our plates. Again, placing large platters of food conveniently on the table is a traditional celebration of our blessings, but is a sword placed to the throat of someone struggling with excess weight.

A second sociological trap is the desire to be elsewhere. When I was in the Navy in Japan, we lived some distance away from the hospital, and rush hour commuting could take three hours to drive the eight miles. By arriving early and working through the lunch hour, I could finish my work, give the Navy a full eight hours, and still leave by three to beat the rush hour traffic. In that way, I could be home in less than an hour, and save about four hours a day commuting. In fact, Navy rules allowed and encouraged this approach. However, the hospital commanding officer strongly objected to my working through lunch so that I could leave early, leaving me the option of eating lunch or working an extra hour. I chose the worst option, and the result was at least ten pounds of weight gain over about eight months. I mention this because eating is a legitimate excuse for leaving your work and taking the break you sorely need, whereas taking a short nap is not socially acceptable. Many people get sick for this same reason: they need rest, and a cold is the only acceptable reason to get what they must have. The body is ingenious in getting its needs met, and if it must play a trick on you, then play a trick it will. The intelligent person will not force his subconscious into deceptive tactics to save his hide. For a busy physician, his patients will accept the fact that he has to eat, they will not accept the fact that he needs a break. The chances are very good that a lot of meals you eat, especially lunches, are eaten solely as an excuse to get out of the office and have a break. That being the case, you need to look for inventive excuses to take the break you need. A lunchtime exercise program at the YMCA, or a fitness center, may serve the same purpose. A brisk walk to the library or the barber may also suffice. In resetting behavior patterns you must become downright ingenious. But you may have to keep your activities secret.

Having explored how the appetite is produced, let us turn to how it is satisfied, since once you have triggered your appetite it will have to be satisfied. Any appetite can be eliminated by activity in another direction. It won't go away by trying to wait it out, because you will dwell on it mentally and it will grow stronger. You are inventive enough to find solutions to that problem. But what if you want to satisfy your appetite without gaining weight? Appetite is satisfied by psychological and physiological factors. Among the physiological factors are an increase in blood sugar and fats, and the volume of food in the stomach. Psychological factors include pleasant surroundings during the meal, what most of us call "atmosphere," and the taste and aroma of food. The actual act of chewing food is both psychologically and physiologically satisfying. In that regard, soft highly processed foods (liquid diet products) do not satisfy the need to chew. Chewing not only stimulates salivation, it improves the health of the teeth and jaws, and prepares the stomach for digestion. (Chewing gum deceives the stomach, preparing it for a sham meal. Chewing gum before or after a meal might be beneficial, however.)

For carbohydrates, most of the digestion occurs in the mouth, and if the food is not properly chewed it is not properly digested. It takes time for blood sugar and lipid levels to rise after a meal, and until it does your appetite will be unabated. If you wolf your food down in five minutes, you will have eaten far too much before your appetite is satisfied. There are several ways you can use these facts to your advantage. A simple way is to eat a fruit appetizer about twenty minutes before the actual meal. By the time the meal is set, your appetite is much reduced. A fruit or vegetable salad will serve the same function, and the oil in the dressing will also help quell the beast within. In fact, so will candy, but carbohydrates have another problem which will be discussed later.

A second way is to slow down the meal process. Slowly chewing each bite will not only slow your eating, but will improve your digestion and satisfy your need to chew. This effect can be bolstered by setting your eating utensils aside while chewing, instead of holding them poised to attack the next morsel. The discipline of setting the eating utensils aside while chewing and contemplating the food being eaten is remarkably effective in reducing the amount of food eaten. You will have to try it to believe it, and the results will be astounding. Water is essential for digesting food, especially proteins and fats. Perhaps as much as a half liter of water is needed to digest a meal, and this water must come from somewhere. You can either drink it with the meal, or let your digestive system take it out of your body fluids. By drinking a full glass of water a few minutes before your meal, and another during the meal you will not only supply the necessary water, but provide volume which will suppress your appetite and also slow your meal, further suppressing your appetite.

How often have you eaten and then not even remembered either that you had eaten or what you had eaten? This is because you were distracted by other activities: reading, conversation, the radio, or TV. By not paying attention to the food, its flavor, appearance, and texture, you were missing a powerful psychological partner for appeasing your appetite. If you have an appetite to eat, then it must be satisfied by the knowledge that you have eaten. By allowing distractions (including family arguments), you will consume a lot more than you intended. You only taste food while it is in your mouth, so keep it there as long as possible to savor its variety.

Volume will also tend to satisfy the appetite, or at least will prevent your eating any more. Non-processed foods rich in fiber will fill the volume faster than highly processed foods. In this regard, fruit and vegetables are ideal. Water also provides volume, and no calories. In fact, the recommended two liters of water a day will require sixty-five calories just warming it to body temperature.

So by eating high fiber foods requiring chewing, you satisfy the need to chew, provide volume to appease your appetite, and allow time for your blood sugar and lipid levels to come to your rescue.

Once satisfied, your appetite will eventually return. A proper diet will forestall that event. Obviously, it is important to avoid those appetite-inducing factors mentioned above. Certain foods will delay the return of your appetite longer than other foods. Carbohydrates, for example, are almost instantly digested to glucose with minimal energy cost, and immediately enter the blood stream where the body must quickly move it into the cells for storage. This requires insulin and chromium. A meal relatively rich in carbohydrates will stress this mechanism severely, with the result that too much insulin will be produced and blood sugar levels will drop to below normal within a hour after eating. This low blood sugar will then stimulate your appetite prematurely. Excess carbohydrates are bad for two reasons, first they are digested with a minimal energy cost, and second the rebound effect just mentioned. Note, however, that you must ingest a minimum of 400 calories as carbohydrate daily or your body will have to burn needed protein in order to stay alive. Carbohydrates should be as unrefined as possible or practical.

Fats require almost as many calories to digest as they produce, and also take so long to digest that they suppress the appetite for a long time. Unfortunately, fats are easily oxidized into toxic by-products and produce malodorous compounds when they are burned for energy. The body is not designed to survive solely off fat. When you are losing weight, incidentally, you are on a high fat diet, because you are consuming yourself. Limit the total number of calories from fat to about 25 percent of your total caloric consumption. Incidentally, when you add the 400 calories obligated to carbohydrates, plus the 180 obligated to protein, and the 20 percent which should be fat, you get a minimum of about 775 calories needed daily. Most commercial crash diets do not provide this, and some do not provide even half this. Such diet plans will cause serious damage, even death.

Proteins also require a fairly high energy expenditure to digest, and also suppress the appetite for a long time. However, once you have provided for all the protein your body needs for the day, the surplus will be converted to sugar (glucose) and burned as energy. If the amount of glucose is excessive, it will be converted to glycogen or fat for storage. When protein is converted to glucose, urea as a by-product must be washed out of the system. This requires water, and lots of it. Most of us are drinking much less than the optimum two liters per day; in fact, some of us hardly touch the stuff. Yet it is the stuff of life itself.

Physical activity results not only in calories burned, but in decreased appetite, so that physical activity should be a part of any weight reduction program. Physical activity engaged in shortly after a meal will result in more calories burned than the same activity done before a meal, but is more stressful to someone out of condition. Excess calories eaten at breakfast results in a more active day, and less weight gain. Eaten at night, the same extra calories will almost always result in weight gain. Skipping breakfast to lose weight is the worst thing you can do. If you must skimp on your meal, do your skimping at the evening meal. A good substitute for the evening meal is a meal consisting of soybean protein supplemented with methionine and fiber to make it a nutritionally complete meal. Notice that no liquid diet product will satisfy the need to chew, nor the psychological input that lets us know that we have truly eaten a meal. Several otherwise acceptable products are available.

Smokers are very inefficient in the use of calories, so that much of what they eat is wasted. Smoking also affects taste, and this results in less food being eaten. When the smoker stops smoking, he is hit with a triple whammy: his taste returns so that food tastes good again; calories are again used efficiently, so that he needs less food than before; and, the nervousness caused by withdrawal is often met by eating. Most former smokers gain several pounds within a few weeks of stopping.

The human body was designed to withstand prolonged periods without food without permanent damage. Whenever we stop eating, we go through a day or two of hunger, then our appetite is subdued until we eat heartily for several consecutive meals. Some years ago, it occurred to me that when the wolf makes a kill, it must eat until all the meat is gone lest the food spoil, then it likely will have to do without food for several days, or perhaps even weeks. That being the case, it is unlikely that God would have created the wolf to be constantly hungry and miserable, but would have created some mechanism to avoid hunger when no food was available. Likewise, when a kill is made, the hunger mechanism must be turned back on by the food so that all the food is eaten and not wasted. In a world in which life depends upon sacrifice of the living, some compensation is necessary. Our God is compassionate to the wolf as well as to the animal killed for food. In the case of the animal being killed, the brain releases powerful narcotic compounds which eliminate pain. In the case of the wolf, a few days without food stops the pangs of hunger.

These facts should prove useful in weight control. Experience proves that a heavy meal is followed by a quick return of hunger. How many times have you raided the kitchen within an hour of eating a feast? Quit feeling guilty: that appetite was as natural as breathing. It is the same mechanism that keeps the wolf from wasting its kill. In your case, however, you waist it. If you think back on your battle of the bulge, you will notice that weight gain came in spurts. Each spurt was initiated by a heavy meal, and continued until the overabundant supply of food ran out.

Here, again, a little knowledge of the compassion of God comes in handy. The eating of a single meal will not bring back the appetite suppressed by days of fasting. It takes several heavy meals to bring back the voracious appetite that puts on weight. In my experience, three heavy meals are required. If I can follow a heavy meal with a very light meal, the return of the beast can be averted. Here, limited calorie meals of the various weight control programs come to the rescue. It is a good way to wean off your addiction.

Most overweight people have known precious few days without hunger because they have fed their appetite. The appetite created by overeating *cannot* be satisfied, it will continue to torment you with hunger until you eat. And then torment you again within an hour of eating. It is an addiction.

The only solution is to use your will power to break the vicious cycle. It takes about two days of fasting to break a gluttonous appetite. The first day will be difficult regardless of what method you use. During that day, the body must adjust to moving food out of storage rather than putting fat into storage. You have about a two-day's supply of immediately convertible carbohydrate stored as glycogen in the liver. After that, you must start burning fat. During the two-day transition period, you will experience nausea, hunger pangs, and perhaps some weakness. Many toxic substances are fat soluble, and are stored in body fat. As this fat is broken down during the diet, these toxic substances are released into the system, and may cause headache and other uncomfortable feelings. Since it is entirely possible to be addicted to food, these feelings can also be due to withdrawal from your addiction. Fortunately, this usually lasts only a day or two. These symptoms can be reduced by drinking fruit juice during the fast. My recommendation is to fast except for fruit juice the first day, then shift over to a soybean nutritional supplement (be sure it is bolstered with methionine, vitamins, minerals, and fiber) the next day. By the third day your metabolism will have made the transition, and you will feel great without hunger or weakness.

The uncomfortable transitional period may be due to withdrawal from the effects of an addictive food allergy. Certain allergic food reactions release narcotic substances from the brain, and these substances are addictive. Long distance runners have the same problem since strenuous exercise releases the same compounds.

If you are able to avoid the voracious appetite that consumes everything within sight, you can fast a single day and feel almost no symptoms of distress. One way to avoid that voracious appetite is to fast regularly. The Biblical admonition to fast one day a week would not only control your appetite, but would eliminate about 3000 calories per week for the average person. It may, in fact, be an ideal weight control program. Three thousand calories translates into 333 grams of fat, or one kilogram of body weight (since fatty tissue is still about two-thirds water). Thus fasting one day a week would probably result in a weight loss of about two pounds a week. In addition, it would release about three hours for other pursuits. The weight loss would be less as you approached your ideal weight.

The satiated feeling that comes with chronic overeating may be due to food allergy or food addiction. The food allergy in turn is frequently the result of Candida albicans overgrowth. The overgrowth is largely the result of our chronic antibiotic intake (antibiotics are in much of our food, especially poultry and beef), and our diet of highly refined carbohydrates which tend to encourage Candida overgrowth. Hormones and birth control pills also aggrevate the situation.

Once your diet is in full swing, you will need to meet nutritional minimums, or you will do harm to your body. A certain amount of undernutrition may be desirable, however. Animal studies have demonstrated that animals underfed in terms of calories and protein, but generously fed in terms of vitamins and minerals, live much longer than usual. Your body is designed for frequent periods without food. When the food supply is greatly diminished, the body in its wisdom will begin to eliminate those older and dying cells first. Eventually, younger cells will also be lost, and this is certainly no good. But the elimination of dying cells is a distinct advantage, because the body is able to function much better without those cells around. During a juice fast, after the initial day or two of misery you will begin to feel much better than you remember ever feeling. This feeling of euphoria will last perhaps two weeks before the lack of protein starts damaging young cells. Before that occurs, you need to begin eating highly nutritious food, minus the extra calories if you still need to lose weight.

At this point the rules of the game are distinctly changed. If you break the rules, you may suffer severe and permanent damage. You must take in at least 400 calories as carbohydrate, plus 45 grams of high quality protein (another 180 calories). If your protein source is incomplete, as is the case of most vegetable proteins, you will have to increase this value significantly, and will get additional calories in the process. If the vegetables eaten are varied you will get a complete amino acid mixture. Depending upon one vegetable type will almost invaribly result in an amino acid deficiency. Most vegetables are deficient in lysine, for which soybeans are an excellent source. Soybeans are deficient in methionine. Additionally, you will need ample potassium and those vitamins necessary for health. Choline will help in the mobilization of fat. Lecithin is an excellent source of choline, but all available processed lecithin is very high in lipid peroxides, which should be avoided. Whole soybeans would be an excellent source of lecithin and choline. If you lack carbohydrate, your body will continue to burn muscle to supply glucose for the brain. Since mobilization of fat will result in high blood lipid levels, increase your vitamin C intake to keep the cholesterol more soluble, and speed its elimination. Fruit juice is again useful here. Be sure to include enough fiber to prevent constipation and also to help eliminate the extra toxic peroxidized cholesterol.

Overeating can also be due to a lack of trace elements. When your body is deficient in any nutrient, it appears to be constantly screaming for more food. Some trace elements are absolutely essential for life, and the fat that comes with getting it is less a danger than being short of essentials. This effect has been proven in the case of iron deficiency, and probably works with other deficiencies as well. Here, a completely balanced meal will result in less food eaten. This is why your diet supplement should contain generous amounts of vitamins and minerals.

If you remember the wolf, you can probably lose weight without difficulty, and without pain. The rules are simple: 1) It one or two days of fasting (taking juice only) to transform your appetite and metabolism to losing weight rather than storing fat. 2) For about one or two weeks after that, you can continue with a juice fast. Your body will eliminate its unhealthy cells to maintain the young healthy ones. This is not mandatory, but is a good practice at least annually to purge the body. 3) Until you reach your desired weight, a diet program for three meals a day (five days a week), or taken for two out of three meals, can be followed indefinitely. An extra tall glass of fruit or vegetable juice daily is recommended. 4) Three heavy meals will restart the appetite cycle. Don't do it! 5) One heavy meal will pose no difficulties if you fast the next meal, drinking only juice. You can prepare for a planned heavy meal by a short juice fast. 6) If you feel satiated, you probably have overeaten. Substitute a low calorie meal for your next meal or two until you again feel the vigor that comes with a reduced caloric intake.

Don't eat unless you are hungry. This should be obvious, but the truth is that most of our meals are eaten because it is there before us. So don't eat without asking yourself if you are hungry. If you're not, then skip the meal and do something constructive.

Food eaten at supper will more likely result in weight gain. If you are going to eat a normal or heavy meal, make it breakfast or lunch. If you plan to use a low calorie product diet plan for only one meal daily, it should be for the evening meal. If two meals are to be substituted, let them be breakfast and supper.

Exercise will actually suppress an abnormal appetite. If you are short of calories, exercise will result in a hearty appetite. But for most of us, regular exercise will result not only in reduced appetite, but much better health. Dieting without exercise is not recommended. Walking probably is the best all around exercise, but there are ample alternatives. A jogging trampoline can be used indoors without regard to the weather, and provides more training benefit in a given period of time than does jogging outdoors, and with less trauma to the feet and knees. A high quality treadmill will make it possible to calibrate your exercise level more precisely, but will cost about $500. Gardening can also fill the bill.

Since we all want a simple formula to go by, let me make this suggestion. 1) Drink at least eight glasses of water daily. 2) Eat at least four servings (one half cup) of vegetables daily, preferably steamed or raw. Microwave cooking is an ideal way to cook vegetables. Two should be yellow vegetables, and one should be of the cabbage family (broccoli, cabbage, cauliflower, brussels sprouts). 3) Eat up to four servings of fresh fruit daily. If only canned fruit is available, pour off the syrup and rinse under water to remove the excess sugar. 4) Your diet should include two pats of butter (*not* margarine) daily. 5) You will need one serving of a whole grain cereal daily, either hot, dry, or in bread. Avoid those with added sugar, salt, or vitamins. You are already getting too much sugar and salt, and you can take your own vitamins more cheaply. 6) Consume two glasses of skim milk or yogurt daily to get needed calcium and protein. 7) Your need for protein will be provided by eggs (boiled, poached, or sunny side up only), meat, cottage cheese, cheese, or legume foods (beans, lentils, or soybeans). Eggs cooked with the yolk membrane intact are wholesome and do not contribute to increased blood LDL cholesterol (the bad kind). Cooked scrambled or in an omelet the yolk cholesterol oxidizes to the toxic peroxidized cholesterol. 8) I strongly recommend a supplemental vitamin/mineral tablet providing nutrients similar to those mentioned later in this book. 9) Certain vegetables should be used often: onion and garlic, peppers, beans, (various types, mixed), asparagus, vegetables of the cabbage family, and soy beans.

Supplements which encourage fat metabolism include Evening primrose oil, Black currant seed oil, Black walnuts, L-Carnitine, lecithin, and all of the "B" vitamins, and Coenzyme Q10.

VI.
Hypertension

Hypertension is a disease in which the blood pressure is elevated beyond acceptable levels. It afflicts a very large percentage of our population, and contributes significantly to premature death. Hypertension is not to be taken lightly. It can seldom be detected without examination, and the first symptoms of its presence may be fatal. Most afflicted with this disease can avoid the serious complications with a combination of drugs, exercise, diet, and routine examinations. If you have not had a routine physical examination or blood pressure check within the past year, I urge you not to neglect your health further.

Each doctor will have a different figure for what pressures he feels are reasonable, based on his experience. Diagnosis and treatment of hypertension should be left to your physician. However, once your pressure is under good control, your physician may recommend your purchasing one of the several accurate monitoring devices available to save some of his time and your money. If you get such a device, be sure to spend enough to get one that is easy to put on and use. Some are rather difficult to use, and may cause your pressure to rise in frustration. This will not eliminate all visits to your doctor, however, since others factors are involved.

In general, the systolic pressure (indicated by the first number) should be between 100 and 120. However, higher pressures may be acceptable in a given situation. The diastolic pressure (indicated by the second number) represents the lowest the blood pressure drops between beats of the heart. It should be between 50 and 80, although up to 90 is accepted as normal. Be aware, however, that even modest elevations of pressure are associated with an increased risk of stroke, myocardial infarction, and death. The higher the blood pressure, the harder the heart must work to pump blood through the networks of blood vessels that supply nutrition and oxygen to the body. Also, the higher the pressure, more fluid will leak out of the vessels, producing edema. Edema, in turn, reduces the amount of oxygen and nutrients supplied to the body, further compromising the function of the blood system and increasing the activity of free radicals.

To better understand what is happening when the heart beats, think of the blood vessels as large rubber tubes. Each time the heart beats, the tubes stretch to absorb the extra volume. The more the tubes stretch, the more blood they can hold, and the less pressure necessary to empty the heart during the contraction. As soon as the heartbeat is over, the tubes begin to contract, emptying the extra volume of blood. As the surplus blood is squeezed out into the peripheral vessels, the pressure is kept from dropping too low by the elasticity of the blood vessels. This elasticity, incidentally, is related to silicon in the diet, and the absence of free radical activity. If the aorta (the main artery fed directly by the heart) is very elastic, it will stretch quickly and prevent the systolic pressure from rising very high. And the large volume of blood it holds while distended serves also to keep the difference between the systolic and diastolic pressures minimal. A wide pulse pressure indicates rigid, hardened arteries. A narrow pulse pressure indicates soft, elastic arteries.

If the peripheral circulation restricts blood flow, then both the diastolic and systolic pressures will be high. The peripheral circulation may be restricted because of poor physical condition (exercise opens many capillary channels in the muscles), anxiety and stress (which causes constriction of capillaries), and certain metabolic and organic diseases which we will not cover here. If blood pools in the veins, called venous stasis, then it acts as a barrier to blood flowing smoothly through the system, just as a swamp slows the flow of water to the sea. Venous stasis is usually the result of too little physical activity, since the major veins are pumps which use muscle activity to pump blood back to the heart. In fact, these major veins do a major portion of the work of pumping blood in active people, taking a major burden off the heart. They are so effective, in fact, that isometric exercises done three times a day will significantly lower blood pressure in many.

Thus, a high systolic pressure associated with a normal diastolic pressure would suggest hardening of the arteries. If both are high, and the pulse pressure is low, then the arteries are okay, but something is increasing peripheral resistance. Actual diagnosis and treatment should be done with the full cooperation of your physician.

Assuming you either have or wish to avoid hypertension, what should you do to lower your blood pressure? If drugs are prescribed, give them a decent trial, and work with your physician to find a combination that will work for you with minimal side effects. However, for most hypertensives, the common sense holistic approach discussed below will work better than any available drug, or at the very least will allow you to be under control with less medication. Different factors are discussed below: apply them as they fit your situation.

WEIGHT. It goes without saying that obesity is associated with hypertension, just as it is associated with an elevated cholesterol. Obesity is also associated with a lot of other ills, so get serious about getting your weight down. The reason why obesity has such a bad track record is related to inactivity and free radical pathology. If you know your problem and refuse to face it squarely, you are telling me you are committing suicide the slow way. Enough said.

SALT. Sodium may not be the bugaboo it is claimed to be, although most of us are consuming thirty times our minimum daily requirement. Certainly, a high sodium intake is associated with hypertension. But many with a high sodium intake have normal pressures. Apparently, some persons respond to a high salt intake with hypertension. Others do not. There is no simple test to distinguish the two groups of people. In any case, we only need about 300 milligrams of sodium daily, and most of us are getting about 10,000 milligrams daily. Since excess salt causes excess fluid retention, it is logical that a sodium excess might cause hypertension.

However, even more important than excess sodium may be our relative potassium deficiency. That is, the ratio of potassium to sodium in the diet is very important, and that ratio has been more than reversed in recent decades. Over the past few decades we have eliminated the rich sources of potassium and substituted processed foods which are usually rich in sodium. Potassium, in sufficient quantities, acts both as a diuretic and anti-hypertensive. It should be remembered that magnesium is essential in the pump mechanism that moves potassium across the cell membrane to the inside of each cell, where it is needed. Thus a magnesium deficiency will result in an intracellular potassium deficiency, and also increased loss of potassium through the kidneys. This is more than academic: magnesium deficiency is very common, if not virtually universal, and has recently been proven to be a major factor in digitalis toxicity generally attributed to potassium deficiency. Thus it requires more than potassium to correct a

44

potassium deficiency. In addition, diets deficient in essential fatty acids (destroyed in the processing of food, and especially in the hydrogenation of oils) result in defective cell membranes that leak sodium into the cells, and leak potassium out. Calcium and magnesium displacement also occurs.

The best sources of potassium are vegetables and fruit, preferably eaten raw; but if cooked, eaten with the juice. Potassium is highly water soluble and will end up in any water used in cooking foods. Meats, generally, are rich in both potassium and sodium. This may be one reason why the vegetarian diet is usually effective in lowering blood pressure.

CAFFEINE is a potent stimulant that increases the pulse rate and constricts blood vessels, both effects which serve to increase blood pressure. To someone not accustomed to caffeine, the effect of caffeine is dramatic, and lasts for at least six hours. During this period, the person is nervous and irritable. When the effect of the caffeine wears off, the nervous system seems to crash leaving the person exhausted and sleepy. If you are a chronic consumer of caffeine, then when the effect wears off you may develop a severe headache, one withdrawal symptom of caffeine addiction or dependance. The hypertensive patient will do well to discontinue all products containing caffeine, including coffee, tea, cola and other carbonated drinks (read the label), and chocolate. When I discontinued regular use of coffee I found I was very sensitive to caffeine, and could only drink about a half cup. Later, when I began taking magnesium, I lost that sensitivity.

SMOKING and TOBACCO products are absolutely out for the hypertensive patient. Smoking one cigarette constricts blood vessels and reduces peripheral circulation by as much as two-thirds for several hours. The anoxia produced enhances free radical pathology and increases the risk of thromboembolic diseases, including stroke, heart attack, thrombophlebitis, and pulmonary emboli. In addition, tobacco smoke contains many free radical catalysts such as complex hydrocarbons and heavy metals, especially cadmium, a known cause of hypertension. Finally, smoking reduces the effeciency of the lungs, compounding all the other problems caused by smoking. Only the last problem is avoided by use of snuff or chewing tobacco, but the risk of oral cancer is increased. The jesting name of "coffin nails" is a bad joke at best, but very true. Tobacco use is addicting, but there is now available (by prescription) nicotine chewing gum which will help wean you off your addiction. Dilantin, 100 milligrams three times a day (also a prescription drug), can also help you overcome the withdrawal pains. Incidentally, it has been calculated that if enough tax were added to the cost of each pack of cigarettes to cover the cost of medical care for associated diseases, and the cost of houses burned down (a very significant figure), the tax would have to be $3.50 per pack. Non-smokers are having to share that burden through increased health care and fire insurance premiums, plus Medicare costs. I realize that the tobacco farmer would be in dire straits without tobacco income, but the cost to the nation far outweighs that income. Regional cooperative alcohol fuel distilleries might be able to partially offset the income loss, especially if such fuel were not taxed.

FOOD ALLERGIES, and Candida albicans induced reactions can produce episodes of elevated blood pressure. Candida overgrowth is a frequent cause of food allergy, by a complex mechanism. The treatment is suspicion and use of drugs to kill the yeast cells within the body, then adjusting the diet to discourage their return.

LIGHT should not be overlooked as a cause of hypertension. Artificial light, deficient in ultraviolet and blue light, has been shown to promote tumor growth, and also hyperactivity in children. Distinct muscle weakness develops instantly upon exposure to artificial light. The duration of labor before delivery and birth is distinctly longer when the birthing rooms use artificial light (as almost all do). Many chemical reactions are catalysed by light, including the beneficial conversion of cholesterol to vitamin D. Many food dyes added prolifically to foods are acted on by light, to produce pharmacologically active compounds. Light passes through our bodies, a fact easily proven by inserting a lighted flashlight into your mouth, and reacts with our body chemistry in both beneficial and harmful ways. A tanned skin is one way in which the body seeks to control the amount of light that penetrates into its interior. Artificial lights corrected to sunlight are available and should be used in work and living areas. Dura-Test is a pioneer in color corrected lighting.

VITAMINS should not be neglected. Niacin, up to 100 milligrams a day, dilates blood vessels and improves circulation. Other vitamins work to reduce the effects of free radicals. In short, I strongly recommend vitamin and trace element supplementation.

WATER is one of the best, and certainly the cheapest diuretic. Whereas we should be drinking two to three liters of water daily, most of us consume less than one liter. Without water, the kidneys cannot get rid of the extra sodium in our diet. In fact, about one liter of water is required just to get rid of the excess salt in our diet, not to mention toxic metabolic wastes. I am not aware of any study proving it, but I suspect that water would be an effective treatment for mild to moderate hypertension. In order to protect the overly enthusiastic, I must warn you that water in excess can deplete the body of sodium and produce coma or death. Limit your water intake to about three liters per day. The hypertensive patient should consider water as an essential medicine, and religiously drink a minimum of two liters (about eight full glasses) a day. Incidentally, water is water, and only water is water. Other liquids, such as tea or soft drinks, also contain chemicals which require water for their removal. Therefore, only water should be counted for the two liters daily. Because chlorine is a potent catalyst of free radicals, I would advise removing the chlorine by allowing the water to set overnight in an open jar (in the refrigerator), or by installing a filter for that purpose on your water faucet. Distilled water can also be used, but is much more expensive.

EXERCISE. Too often we think that only the heart pumps blood. Actually, the body has many pumping stations, and the heart is just the major one. All of the veins in your limbs have valves which allow blood flow in one direction only: back toward the heart. Every time you tighten your muscles, you are pumping blood back to the heart, and away from the periphery. If you are physically inactive, blood pools in your arms and legs. The heart must pump harder to move this stagnant blood around and back to the heart again. The result is elevated blood pressure. Every time you exercise you are pumping blood back to the heart and taking a load off the heart, and thereby lowering your blood pressure. The venous pump, as it is called, is so effective that merely tensing your muscles and holding them tense for six seconds three times daily results in a considerable reduction in blood pressure within a few weeks! The current fad of hanging upside down is designed to ease stagnant pooling of blood. It certainly does that. However, there are no valves in the veins above the heart, and blood pools in the head while one is hanging by his heels. I would rather have stagnant blood in my legs than in my head, especially if I had a weak blood vessel inside my skull. Varicose veins in your legs look terrible but a ruptured blood vessel inside your head can kill you.

Even more effective than isometric exercises is a more strenuous exercise program. To be maximally effective, the exercise should last for at least twelve minutes each time, although thirty minutes would be even better. It should be sufficient to cause the heart to beat faster, preferably pushing the heart rate to 150 beats per minute for twelve minutes or more, but this should not be done without the consent of your physician, and prior preparation and a conditioning program. If you go at it gung-ho without gradually building your stamina, you will become sore and discouraged. And you will quit the exercise program. Worse, your poor condition will result in severe anoxia, which will produce many free radicals, which *may* trigger a thrombosis in rather inconvenient places. From that you may die. So start slowly with a conditioning program, remembering that you are building for the long haul, namely the rest of your life, and you will be glad when each day finds you a bit stronger than you were the day before. There are several excellent exercise programs available, and excellent books written. Pick one that fits your situation and stick with it. Exercise is most effective, and much safer, if it is entered into with a warmup period, and ended with a cooling off period of several minutes. Warmup, exercise, cooling off, and a quick shower should take only about thirty minutes, and will add several times that to your day in improved efficiency and a reduced need for sleep. That gain in time is not to mention the probable increase in productive lifespan, which may run into years. Such an exercise program, performed at least thrice weekly, will improve and maintain your overall physical condition. Incidentally, exercise produces lactic acid, which is an effective chelating agent with all the benefits of chelation. Chelation acts by removing toxic lipid peroxide catalysts such as ionic iron and copper, so that free radical pathology is checked and the body can begin the healing process of reversing atherosclerosis. It is not true that athletes do not develop atherosclerosis, they most certainly do, and do so as rapidly as the rest of us. But those who are vigorously active develop larger blood vessels and thus avoid some of the dangers of atherosclerosis. The key to preventing atherosclerosis is dietary control of free radical pathology, plus judicious use of chelation therapy, and intelligent use of thyroid hormone.

GARLIC and ONION both reduce fat droplets in the blood, and also tend to dilate blood vessels. There is good evidence that these two herbs will lower blood pressure, and blood cholesterol, eaten regularly. They contain potent antioxidants, and are therefore effective against free radicals. Both are effective when cooked, and are certainly less offensive when cooked. Both have been shown to be effective for about 40 percent of hypertensives within a few weeks of their daily use. Garlic and onion should be eaten especially with fatty meals. Deodorized garlic oil is available commercially, and retains the benefits of garlic.

CADMIUM TOXICITY is a known cause of hypertension. And

cadmium is by-product of modern civilization. It is used to plate metals to prevent rusting and shows up almost everywhere. In addition, cadmium is present in tobacco smoke in sufficient quantities to produce toxicity. Disposal of worn out nickel-cadmium batteries in landfills may contribute to an increase in cadmium in the water supply, and is a problem that needs to be addressed immediately. Fortunately, the toxic effects of cadmium can be reduced by increasing your zinc intake. Limit zinc to about 45 milligrams, however, otherwise you risk inducing copper deficiency by zinc competition with copper. Zinc itself is safe in doses of up to 60 milligrams per day. However, if your water supply is soft or acidic, and your plumbing copper, there is a strong possibility that you are already getting too much copper, and are suffering from copper toxicity. In that case, zinc may reduce your copper toxicity. A second way of getting rid of cadmium is by taking vitamin C, four to six grams daily. Vitamin C is a poor man's chelation therapy: it's slow, but it works. Chelation itself is very effective in removing cadmium and other toxic heavy metals.

CALCIUM DEFICIENCY also seems to produce hypertension. When the heart contracts, or an artery contracts to increase the "tone," calcium passes through "channels" in the muscle cell walls to cause the contraction. If it were possible to block some of these channels, it would be possible to lower blood pressure. For this reason, the medical profession is justly excited about calcium channel blockers recently introduced to lower blood pressure. It would seem that taking more calcium would simply aggravate the situation, and force an increase in blood pressure. As all too often, the obvious is not true. Calcium deficiency increases the activity of the parathyroid gland, resulting in more ionized calcium in the blood, which in turn results in more calcium being available to pass through those channels. Supplemental calcium suppresses the activity of parathyroid hormone, which reduces the amount of ionized calcium in the blood and thus acts like a calcium channel blocker.

Calcium supplements have been successfully used in treatment of hypertension. One gram daily was used, and was effective within six weeks.

MAGNESIUM DEFICIENCY is also associated with hypertension, and is quite common. Magnesium injections are used to control severe hypertension of pregnancy (ecclampsia), an effective treatment known for well over a decade. It has been known for many years that heart disease is less common where the water is hard (the result of magnesium salts). Whereas calcium causes the heart muscle to contract strongly, magnesium is necessary for relaxation of muscle. Magnesium is also important for anyone taking calcium, since the ratio of magnesium to calcium in the diet is important. Taking calcium without also taking magnesium increases your risk of kidney stones, cardiovascular diseases, and abnormal calcium deposits throughout the body. Magnesium works as a co-factor with pyridoxine (B6), and is depleted when very high doses of pyridoxine is taken. Taken with pyridoxine, magnesium is effective in preventing kidney stones, even when supplemental calcium is also taken.

Recently, I had a patient who had a hemorrhage in his eye, and in the course of taking a medical history he told me that his blood pressure had not been below 200/140 in five years, in spite of the best efforts of several physicians. His diet was deficient in vitamins and minerals. I took his blood pressure, 220/144, and put him on supplements equivalent to that listed later in this book. One week later his blood pressure was 150/104. Still high, but remarkably lower. I believe that magnesium deficiency was his primary problem.

Magnesium is the essential metal in the enzyme pump that pumps vital potassium into cells. Without potassium, cells, especially heart muscle, do not function properly. Magnesium deficiency is now proven to be important in digitalis toxicity previously thought to be due in part to potassium deficiency. Since without magnesium, potassium cannot enter cells, potassium will be lost to the body if there is a magnesium deficiency. Digitalis toxicity has resulted in the premature deaths of many people, so do not think that magnesium deficiency is benign: it can kill you.

A VEGETARIAN DIET is also effective in lowering blood pressure. The reasons may be manifold: improved potassium/ sodium ratio, increased magnesium, reduced fat consumption and thus fewer free radicals, reduced calories, lower iron consumption (and thus fewer free radicals), and reduced protein. When we consume more protein than we need for health, we burn the rest for energy or convert it to fat. In the conversion of amino acids (from which protein is made) to energy, toxic nitrogen by-products are produced which must be eliminated through the kidneys. The vegetarian diet is relatively poor in the sense that a lot must be consumed to get needed nutrients, including calories. Since there is a limit to how much food a person's stomach can hold, the vegetarian seldom becomes obese. He seldom ingests too much protein (the opposite is more likely the problem), so that toxic products from protein catabolism are not produced. On the plus side, the percentage of calories supplied by fat is greatly reduced. In my own personal experience, I have found that eliminating all animal proteins in my diet results in lowered blood pressure within a few weeks. The effect persists for up to a year for me. Since I have repeated this cycle three times so far, I believe that for me a protein excess is poisonous. However, I have an inherited kidney disease which reduces kidney function and makes this more critical for me. Nevertheless, do not ignore the potential avenue of reducing your excess protein consumption as a means of controlling your blood pressure. It has worked for many.

Magnesium deficiency should be suspected in all cases of potassium deficiency not responsive to therapy, constipation; muscle weakness, twitching, and cramping; angina and irregular heartbeats, slightly elevated calcium levels, mental depression and/or irritability, loss of memory, and tingling sensations. Sensitivity to caffeine may be a sign of magnesium deficiency.

A heart which has stopped beating can frequently be restarted after giving 32 milliequivalents of magnesium chloride intravenously. Magnesium deficiency contributes to the majority of cardiac deaths. And perhaps to other deaths as well, since sudden infant death syndrome (SIDS) is associated with maternal and infant magnesium (and vitamin C) deficiency.

Recent (1986) reports in the literature indicate that persons regularly taking magnesium supplements have only half the risk of having a heart attack. Persons who have had a heart attack and are given magnesium intravenously upon admission to the hospital were 83% less likely to die during that admission.

The ideal magnesium supplement would contain 50 milligrams as magnesium orotate, 50 as the aspartate, and 100 milligrams of potassium as the orotate and aspartate. A reasonable dose would be 1-3 tablets at meals and at bedtime. An overdose would have a laxative effect.

Coenzyme Q10, a totally non-toxic food substance necessary for energy production, will lower blood pressure about 10 points within a few weeks. A recommended dose is 90 to 300 milligrams per day for 3 months, then 30-60 milligrams daily as a maintenance dose.

VII.
Arthritis

From the onset, I would like the reader to understand that I am not an expert in diagnosing nor treating arthritis. Nevertheless, I have become active in treating joint and bone disease somewhat by default. Patients whom I am treating for cataracts began returning, saying that their arthritis pain had stopped. One patient said, "I don't care if my cataracts are better or worse, I am free from pain for the first time in years!" With endorsements like that, who could help but get excited? I can't.

Being a physician whose interests extend beyond the eyes, I have begun treating my patients who also have arthritis. There are several different diseases which are commonly called arthritis by the laity. These need to be distinguished by the physician and patient, since the treatment will be considerably different in each case.

I have a close friend who had been afflicted for several years by arthritis which caused swelling of both ankles. Treatment with all the standard medicines, including gold injections, were ineffective. Finally, he went to a physician who was nutritionally aware, and this physician took him off all foods of the Nightshade family: potato, tomato, tobacco, peppers, and eggplant. The swelling and pain were gone within a few weeks. He remained symptom-free for about two years, when he indulged in some French fries. The swelling developed so quickly he could hardly walk back to the car. Nightshade allergy is one cause of arthritis. Its diagnosis is the result of suspicion. Its treatment is the elimination of foods from that family of plants. Tobacco, of course, is not a food, but it is a member of the nightshade family. Since allergy to tobacco smoke is common, it may be that tobacco is the agent that triggers nightshade allergy. It is a subject worth investigating.

Foods other than members of the nightshade family can and do cause arthritis. Sometimes the allergy is not directly to a specific food, but to a toxic metabolic product from a Candida albicans (a type of yeast) overgrowth in the intestine. Again, the diagnosis is by suspicion, and the elimination of the offending foods. Because of the prevalent, but unrecognized, effect of Candida infections, it would be reasonable to empirically treat for Candida before reinstating foods in a trial situation. In any case, food allergies should be suspected at the onset of treatment for arthritis, and a Candida infection should be suspected as the root cause of the food allergy.

Osteoporosis is a disease of calcium deficiency resulting in reduced mineralization of the bones. If the demineralization is severe, osteomalacia may result, causing pain. I believe that a lot that passes for arthritis is due to calcium and magnesium deficiencies, plus possible silicon deficiency. In any case, the majority of my patients complaining of joint and bone pains find relief by taking calcium, magnesium, and alfalfa. Vitamin D supplements are not necessary because we Americans are already ingesting near-toxic amounts of this vitamin. The alfalfa is a rich source of silicon. (Silicon substitutes for carbon in many tissues, producing stronger molecules, and is necessary for strong bone formation.) Certainly, a large percentage of patients with joint and bone pain will find relief by supplementing their diet with vitamins (especially C, E, and B6), and the minerals calcium, magnesium, and silicon. Phosphorus is also necessary, but usually is a surplus in our diet.

Other causes of arthritis include auto-immunity (when one is allergic to his own body), gout, infection, and inflammation. Gout is a metabolic disease treated with diet and medications. Gout can be caused by some medications, a fact less known.

Inflammation, such as occurs in a joint not accustomed to use, results in acid production, which in turn results in the dissolving of adjacent bone. The calcium crystals are then redeposited in nearby tissues, producing pain. Since magnesium supplements tend to prevent calcium deposits (well proven in the case of kidney stones), magnesium will give relief to patients suffering from arthritis. Incidently, muscle cramps that are not relieved by vitamin E or potassium indicate a magnesium deficiency, magnesium being necessary for proper utilization of both vitamin E and potassium.

Copper is essential in all healing processes, transforming vitamin C into its active forms. In this process, copper is essential to collagen synthesis. Iron and zinc are also involved in the process. However, be aware that both copper and iron, in excess, are potent catalysts for lipid peroxide formation, which, in turn, is one cause of many degenerative diseases, including arthritis. Supplemental

53

copper or iron is not recommended without first testing for iron and copper levels. A serum ferritin test is done for iron, while both hair analysis (done by a reliable laboratory) or erythrocyte copper levels are accurate for copper. Excess iron can be removed easily by donating blood. Excess copper is most easily removed by chelation, or by increasing your zinc consumption. Copper salts pass through the skin in sufficient quantity that some arthritis sufferers benefit from wearing copper bracelets. Aspirin, incidentally, removes copper from the lining of the stomach, and transports it to the areas of inflammation. Aspirin combined with copper is as effective as plain aspirin in relieving inflammation, yet will actually speed the healing of a stomach ulcer. Regular aspirin can be a cause of stomach ulcers.

In one study, half of arthritic patients treated had moderate to excellent improvement on treatment with vitamin A and zinc, both of which are essential to tissue repair. Niacinamide has also been shown to be effective, in high doses, for some victims of arthritis. Silicon, present in the skins of vegetables and bran of cereals, appears to be necessary for proper calcium deposition in bone. Some victims of arthritis respond favorably to silicon therapy. Silicon is also commonly deficient in the modern diet. The so-called "Willard water" touted by its proponents in treatment of arthritis and degenerative diseases is an excellent source of soluble silicon, and apparently also trace minerals. It is made from sodium metasilicate, calcium chloride, epsom salts (magnesium sulfate), and the soluble minerals (probably trace elements) found in lignite, a brown coal between peat and bituminous coal in character. It may act through correction of a silicon and other trace element deficiencies.

A reasonable approach to arthritis would be to determine if mineral or vitamin deficiencies are possible, then supplement accordingly. Suggested supplements include calcium and magnesium, zinc, copper, manganese, iron, silicon (alfalfa is an excellent source), and the vitamins A, C, E, niacin, niacinamide, and B-complex. (Remember, however, the risk of copper and iron toxicity.) One study in England found that some arthritis patients are deficient in pantothenic acid, and respond to pantothenic acid injections. The study suggested that perhaps arthritics cannot absorb the vitamin.

If cortisone or anti-inflamatory drugs are necessary, then vitamin C doses should be increased to several grams daily, since these drugs have been proven to deplete body stores of vitamin C. A recent study done at Georgetown University concluded that vitamin C should always be given with steroid therapy to reduce the harmful side effects of this treatment.

I recently attended a medical conference in which one lecture given by a physician whose practice is primarily in treatment of arthritic patients demonstrated conclusively that 83% of arthritics coming to his clinic were made free of the pain and complications of arthritis by identifying the food to which they were allergic and eliminating that from the diet. Generally only one food was the offending food for a given patient. The eight most common allergens were soy bean, beef, milk products, eggs, tomatoes, potatoes, eggplant, and yeast. Contrary to the more commonly held belief, those allergic to one member of the nightshade family were not really likely to be allergic to other members of that family. Generally, I noted that the most common allergens were those foods which had been introduced to the diet of infants prematurely during the 1950s when breast feeding was being discouraged, and acceleration of the feeding schedule encouraged. Apparently we have created a generation of allergic adults by our deviation from the natural program in the '50s. In conversation after the symposium, this physician told me that in another study, yet unpublished, that about 50 percent of those with allergies were hypothyroid by the Broda O. Barnes' criteria, and had their arthritis relieved upon having thyroid hormone administered.

I believe the explanation for this is that a deficiency in thyroid hormone results in incompletely digested food, and these long chain molecules can be absorbed into the blood stream where they evoke an allergic reaction. Adequate thyroid hormone levels result in more complete digestion, and therefore a reduction in food allergies. I have seen this occur sufficiently often to believe that this is a contributing factor in many arthritic patients.

Also in my experience, the majority of patients with milder forms of arthritis find their pain relieved by the ingestion of a high mineral product such as Body Toddy™ or Spirulina. For these products to relieve the symptoms suggests strongly that mineral deficiencies are an underlying cause of some cases of arthritis.

My main admonition at this point is that arthritis may be due to nutritional deficiencies, food allergy, and/or to intestinal Candidiasis. All three are probably factors with most patients. I believe most cases of arthritis will be found to respond to nutritional therapy once those whose expertise is in arthritis are linked with nutritional knowledge. Certainly, the number of patients whom I have seen improved is an indication that deficiencies are present.

VIII.
Diabetes

Diabetes mellitus is a disease in which the afflicted person cannot handle sugar normally. As a result, blood sugar levels may rise to very high levels causing many problems. Until insulin was discovered, most diabetics died early, and most had no children since the disease is almost incompatible with fertility. After the discovery of insulin, and its availability for therapeutic use, young diabetics began living long enough to have families, and the incidence of the disease has increased.

The increase in diabetes has been greater than can be explained by mere genetics, however, and other factors are obviously at work.

Diabetics fall prey to many vascular and debilitating diseases which are less common in normal individuals. These vascular diseases may develop in spite of therapy with insulin, and may precede the appearance of elevated blood sugars. Some think that diabetics become immune to the animal insulin used, or that an allergic reaction is occurring. Now that the Chinese have unraveled the insulin molecule, and genetic engineers have succeeded in transplanting the gene that produces human insulin into bacteria, human insulin is available in quantity. We will now discover whether immunity to animal insulin is a factor. Certainly, a diabetic should consult with his physician about the possible use of human insulin.

Vascular diseases to which the diabetic is more prone include atherosclerosis, diabetic retinopathy, cataracts, kidney failure due to vascular insufficiency, poor circulation especially in the legs and arms, and poor resistance to infection. As a result, the diabetic can expect a shorter lifespan, and is more likely to suffer blindness, frequent severe infections, and even amputation of limbs. Because of their susceptibility to vascular diseases, the diabetic is strongly advised to quit smoking. The smoking of even one cigarette can reduce blood circulation to the feet and hands by as much as two-thirds, for as long as several hours, compounding the effects of diabetes. It cannot be overemphasized that diabetics should not smoke. Likewise, because exercise both increases circulation and lowers blood sugar, a vigorous exercise program should be the part of the lifestyle of every diabetic.

Dr. Stephen E. Langer, whose book is included in the reading list at the end of this book, cites Broda O. Barnes, M.D., Ph.D., whose work strongly suggests that the vascular problems associated with diabetes are actually the result of subclinical hypothyroidism. Over a period of several decades, both demonstrated that desiccated thyroid will prevent, and even reverse, the vascular complications of diabetes. They recommend a simple test, the Barnes Basal Temperature Test (JAMA 119:1072 August, 1942), which is as reliable as the basal metabolic rate, and is far more reliable than standard laboratory tests. Better yet, it is absolutely free and is done at home. It is performed by measuring the oral temperature immediately upon awakening. The test is repeated for two consecutive days. (The test is not valid during menstruation or fever.) A normal BBTT is 97.8-98.2 degrees F. Anything below that indicates probable hypothyroidism. My preferred treatment is with Cytomel,™ 25-75 mcg daily, adjusting the dosage at 3-day intervals until the BBTT rises toward normal. This becomes the maintenance dose.

These harmful effects of diabetes may be logically related to nutrition. Chromium has been shown to be necessary for the use of insulin, and is also necessary for cardiac and vascular health. Chromium has been proven to stabilize the blood sugar of persons with moderate high and low blood sugar levels. Compounding the problem is the fact that high blood sugar levels cause a loss of chromium from inside body cells into the bloodstream and thus it is lost through the kidneys, so that diabetics are very apt to be deficient in chromium. Since chromium deficiency is very common, even without the effect of diabetes, there can be no justification for the failure to recommend chromium supplements for diabetic patients. However, the solution may not be so simple for severe diabetics, who seem to be unable to convert dietary chromium into the active glucose tolerance factor, known as GTF. For insulin-dependent diabetics, I recommend use of glucose tolerance factor (GTF) instead of chelated chromium. Brewer's yeast is an excellent source of GTF, but has a significant allergic risk. The SeRoyal™ brand seems most effective.

Manganese is also essential for glucose metabolism, and is generally markedly deficient in the average American diet. Diets I have analysed provide less than 1 percent of the amount we probably need. Thus manganese supplementation should be seriously considered.

It has now been proven that vitamin E deficiency can result in diabetic cataracts which are reversible with vitamin E supplementation. In addition, Quercitin, 1000-2000 mg per day, will block the formation of cataracts in diabetics when blood sugar is consistently high. Since magnesium and selenium deficiencies are common, and these minerals are essential for the normal function of vitamin E, their supplementation should also be considered. In fact, a deficiency in antioxidant activity (combined effect of vitamin C, E, and B-complex, plus selenium, zinc, and glutathione) will produce diabetic (as well as other) cataracts. Likewise, these cataracts can be partially or completely reversed by bolstering the antioxidant capacity.

It further appears that vitamin C and glucose (blood sugar) use the same transport system (blood binding molecule), so that the diabetic is handicapped by not being able to effectively move vitamin C to sites of need throughout the body. Since vitamin C is essential in recycling vitamin E in its role as a free radical scavenger, this results in increased free radical pathology for the diabetic. All of the diseases more common in the diabetic are known to be the result of free radical damage.

Assuming you are diabetic, or know someone who is, what should you do? Obviously, every person is different and it would be foolish for me to make a blanket program and expect it to apply to everyone. Certain guidelines will apply, however, and these should be used in cooperation with your family physician.

WEIGHT. Obesity itself contributes to diabetes. Many diabetics would have normal blood sugars if they would discipline themselves sufficiently to get their weight under control. I suggest diabetics study the chapter on weight control carefully. Note that hypothyroidism will make weight control impossible until it is corrected. Fat competes with muscle for insulin—and wins.

EXERCISE. Physical activity causes glucose (blood sugar) to enter cells without the need for insulin. Exercise alone will control blood sugar in many who suffer from mild diabetes. Additionally, exercise improves the health of the heart and blood vessels, major areas of concern for the diabetic. Exercise is also essential for weight control. The diabetic who refuses to trim up and begin a sensible exercise program is committing slow suicide. Since the B-complex vitamins and vitamin E are consumed in exercise, their supplementation is needed.

DIET. Raw vegetables seem to stabilize blood sugar better than do cooked vegetables. Use raw vegetables whenever possible.

Interestingly, the leaves of the blueberry plant, prepared as a tea, will also lower blood sugar. Blueberry leaves, however, will not replace insulin. Sugar should be avoided because it provides calories without chromium, and also depletes body chromium. Avoid all highly processed foods, especially white flour products and white sugar. Needless to say, high fat foods need to be avoided to control weight. Diabetics tend to have increased cholesterol levels in spite of insulin therapy, perhaps in part due to their inability to fully utilize vitamin C, but it has been found that fiber from the "Devil's Tongue" plant, as well as from oats, guar gum, and legumes, will reduce both blood sugar levels and cholesterol, something insulin will not do. Not all fiber is effective, and the effect is thought by some to be due to micronutrients in some types of fiber.

SUPPLEMENTS. Diabetics need those vitamins and minerals which have been proven beneficial to vascular health. These include chromium, copper, manganese, selenium, silicon, zinc, vitamin C, vitamin E, inositol, choline, and bioflavinoids. Vitamin C in large doses has been proven to reduce the amount of insulin required to control insulin dependent diabetics. Since some diabetics cannot convert beta carotenes to vitamin A, the usual result of hypothyroidism, they must include vitamin A from fish liver oils in their diet. Vitamin A is essential in an indirect way for the function of insulin. The combination of an inability to convert beta carotenes, the reduced amount of retinol in the diabetics diet as a result of attempts at weight control (retinol is fat soluble), and the known vitamin A deficiency in the American population in general makes vitamin A supplementation in diabetics mandatory. Zinc is essential for vitamin A to move from its stores in the liver, and vitamin E is essential to protect vitamin A from oxidation into toxic by-products.

Other minerals which may prove to be valuable include vanadium, molybdenum, and tin. We probably are getting enough tin through canned foods, but a vanadium deficiency is probable.

Since diabetics are generally infested with Candida, treatment with anti-yeast drugs plus a daily ration of yogurt with active yogurt culture is advisable. If the yogurt is active the label will display this clearly.

Thyroid therapy is indicated when the Barnes Basal Temperature Test indicates hypothyroidism, as it probably will. (p. 57)

Although this common sense approach will not cure diabetes, it will hopefully make the majority of diabetics free from many of the hazards of the disease, and many will be able to avoid both oral drugs (which increase the risk of heart disease) and insulin injections. I must point out that careful studies in the benefits of the program suggested above have not been made, although known effects and benefits of the nutrients mentioned suggest that the program would be beneficial. Certainly, some elements of the program have been tested and are proven effective. For example, the vascular kidney complications in diabetes responds to nutritional therapy. In my practice, early diabetic retinopathy generally reverses with nutritional therapy. The only risk would be to your finances. I do not believe that the known risk of complications associated with diabetes allows us the luxury of ignoring the potential benefits of nutritional therapy. If you are diabetic, and decide that you will go on a nutritional program, first find a physician who will cooperate, and let him monitor your blood sugar levels and eye fundus appearance carefully as you implement the various nutritional changes. I firmly believe you will be rewarded with improved health, and a longer life.

Supplementation with DMG and Coenzyme Q10 also reduce the need for insulin, and should be tried.

I cannot emphasize too strongly that thyroid function should be tested by the Barnes Basal Temperature Test (BBTT) (see page 57), and if the BBTT is low, treatment with desiccated thyroid or Cytomel™ is essential. I now prefer Cytomel™ because I am finding a fairly large percentage of patients who are apparently unable to convert T4 to T3. Cytomel™ is pure T3. Oral temperatures are equally accurate. Virtually all diabetics are hypothyroid, and this results in an inability to convert beta carotene to vitamin A and retinal. Vitamin A is involved in vision and all healing processes. Chemical tests for hypothyroidism should be done to rule out hyperthyroidism in spite of low body temperature. Quercitin, one of the bioflavinoids, has been proven to prevent formation of cataracts due to elevated blood sugars in diabetics. Also, in a recent study published in Australia, patients receiving vitamin E were 56 percent less likely to develop cataracts than the control group, and patients receiving vitamin C in moderate does were 70 percent less likely to develop cataracts. Since copper or zinc deficiency can produce clinical hypothyroidism with a normal serum level of thyroid hormone, their adequacy should be tested by hair analysis or blood tests. Hair analysis kits may be obtained from Bio-Zoe, Inc., P.O. Box 49, Waynesville, North Carolina 28786.

In addition, all diabetics should have a careful examination by their ophthalmologist at least annually. An ophthalmologist is a physician with specialty training in eye diseases.

IX.
Nutrition and Vision

About the first thing a child learns about nutrition is that he should eat carrots because they are good for his eyes. Needless to say, as an ophthalmologist I am interested in the eyes, and as a physician alert to nutritional problems I do not neglect the eyes. Carrots are good for the eyes, of course, but there is much more to nutrition and vision than carrots.

During the past nine months, I have examined eight children who had loss of vision related to nutrition, the loss being very similar to that seen in alcohol-tobacco amblyopia, although neither alcohol nor tobacco was a factor in any of these children. For the past several years, I have routinely checked children for color vision, stereopsis, and ability to focus at near. These are *not* routine tests, and I know of no other ophthalmologist who does these tests routinely for all children old enough to cooperate. I firmly believe they should be routine.

One of the first signs of vitamin A deficiency is loss of color vision. If a color vision test is not performed the cause will not be discovered early, since only later is there a loss of central vision, accommodation, and stereopsis. Each of the children diagnosed with this problem had similar diet histories: no breakfast (or a high sugar cereal breakfast), a fast food lunch at school (generally chips, a baloney sandwich, and beans), and a fast food supper usually consisting of a hamburger and fries with a soft drink. Most consumed no milk. Only one took any vitamin supplement, and she took one of the simple chewable vitamins pushed in TV advertising.

All except one agreed to nutritional supplementation. And all of those so treated recovered completely within six weeks. The one who refused went to another ophthalmologist who denied that she had a problem. That ophthalmologist did not test for color vision, stereopsis, nor near vision. He did report her vision as 20/25 but said that was normal. (It may be normal, but in view of a loss of color vision within the previous six weeks it was not normal for this child.) I mention this because awareness is the key to diagnosis. Everyone, doctors included, see only what they are trained to see. If you are unaware of nutritional diseases, you will never see them, even when they stare you full in the face.

Incidently, glaucoma is another disease which may appear in children. Current wisdom is that there is no need to test anyone under the age of thirty, because the disease rarely occurs in younger persons. I have several patients with glaucoma who are under thirty, and two who are under ten years of age. The younger ones all had a family history of glaucoma. Therefore, I routinely test for glaucoma in anyone able to cooperate with the test.

People under stress frequently develop a disease called macular edema in which fluid leaks from the vessels behind the eye and forms a pool beneath the retina. During my training in the Washington, D.C., area during the Vietnam War era I saw many in which the pooling formed a large blister beneath the retina. Now that I practice in a small mountain community in western North Carolina, where stress is not so great, I almost never see the disease in this extreme manifestation. But I do still see a milder form, which, unfortunately, is more difficult to diagnose. In both forms vision is adversely affected, sometimes permanently. Since the majority of cases are self-limited and resolve within six weeks, the usual practice is to wait a few weeks before doing anything, then either trying steroids (hormones) or using a laser to seal the leak, if a specific leak can be identified. In 1973, I discovered that by use of vitamin C and bioflavinoids many of these would resolve more rapidly. Resolution was so predictable that when resolution occurred it almost always was on the seventh day. My cure rate using vitamins was better than the published figures using either laser or steroids. I do not claim that the use of vitamin C and bioflavinoids is unique to my practice, for I know of several older ophthalmoloists who successfully use the same combination.

More recently, I have found that some patients with similar symptoms and signs will respond to vitamin E. Note that all three of these vitamins (C, E, and bioflavinoids) are antioxidant, and also have beneficial effects on small blood vessel leakage.

I have discovered the hard way that when a patient comes in with a prescription for glasses that has changed markedly in power (especially toward the plus side), or in astigmatism, then vitamins will not only improve their vision, but will in many cases change their prescription. Therefore, when I suspect swelling in the macular area is the cause of astigmatism or a change in prescription, I do not dispense glasses without first using a two weeks' therapeutic trial of vitamins. In many cases, the prescription changes considerably for the better, and we have avoided the embarrassing problem and expense of changing the glasses again within a few weeks. Needless to say, I don't just use the three specific vitamins now, but take a nutritional history and treat accordingly.

During the past five years, I have seen many patients whose astigmatism gradually decreased over a period of months from as much as five diopters (a very large amount of astigmatism) to as little as one diopter. My Dad's astigmatism came down from 5.5D to 1.25D. My wife's decreased from 4.5D to 1.25D. And I have seen many other cases. The problem, from my point of view, is that it is imperative to explain this to the patient before beginning vitamin therapy, otherwise they return angry that the doctor missed on the prescription. I have wondered how many patients I have seen who switched from their former eye practitioner because their prescription was no longer correct, had caused their own problem by going on vitamins. I know this has been the case in a few patients, whom I assured that their former doctor had not made a mistake. For the discerning reader, I would like to point out that the effect of reducing astigmatism has worked even on patients with corneal astigmatism. I have no idea how it would do that. Apparently, with the proper building materials the eye is able to restructure itself to the proper shape.

Incidentally, there has been one epidemiologic study which indicated that myopia (nearsightedness) is less common in areas where the water supply has ample chromium. It has been clearly shown that myopia is more common today than a generation before. It has also been clearly shown that our diet has shifted away from chromium-rich foods toward those which are not only deficient in chromium, but deplete the body of chromium. I have started children who are beginning to become myopic on a vitamin supplement including chromium, and hopefully will have sufficient data within a few years. In the meantime, use your discretion in regards to your family. Chromium has too many known benefits to omit from a child's diet. I seriously doubt it will reverse myopia already present.

In 1979, I discovered that zinc would reverse certain types of cataracts. It has also been shown that salmon eating a zinc deficient diet develop cataracts. The lens of the eye, in which the cataract develops, is embryologically derived from the same tissue that produces skin. Zinc has been known for years to promote healing of skin diseases. The cataracts most likely to respond to zinc are the cortical cataracts, and those in which there is a milky character to the normally clear cortex. I usually refer to this in my notes as being opalescent. It is not effective for nuclear sclerotic cataracts, nor rapidly effective for posterior subcapsular cataracts. The latter do sometimes respond after a period of many months. If vitamin/mineral therapy is going to work, you will see a response within six weeks, and improvement may continue for a year or more. I have seen vision improve from as bad as 20/200 to 20/20, but the usual improvement is about 50 percent. This is frequently sufficient to avoid surgery.

Other ophthalmologists have discovered that high doses of B-complex is beneficial to cataract patients, and it has been shown that selenium is the active metal in one of the enzyme systems which goes awry during cataract formation. Vitamin C is also extremely important in the lens, perhaps because it scavenges free radicals which would be produced in abundance in the lens because of its exposure to infrared light. The healthy lens has the highest concentration of vitamin C of any tissue of the body; but, vitamin C disappears completely from a cataractous lens. The lens not only focuses light on the retina so that we can see, it is a selective filter removing infrared light so that the retina is not burned by these wavelengths. In the process of stopping these high energy photons, many free radicals would be formed. The high levels of vitamin C in the lens are thought by some to scavenge the free radicals thus formed. A lens exposed to intense sunlight becomes brown, and sometimes this brunescence can be so dense that vision is impaired, and the brunescent cataract must be removed. This brunescence is reversible with antioxidant vitamins, although the reversal is slow and takes many months. Sometimes it is more important to do surgery and restore vision immediately, than it is to wait in blindness the many months necessary for vision to improve. It is a decision requiring an informed patient and surgeon, weighing the costs and options fully.

Some cataracts which did not respond to zinc and B-complex therapy have responded when vitamin E was added to the treatment. This should have been anticipated, since vitamin E and selenium work together, and selenium is important to one of the enzyme systems in the eye. In any case, I had already found that vitamin E benefits vision in those without cataracts, especially in those elderly patients who are more apt to have cataracts. My present practice is to use a potent multivitamin/mineral product which supplies the necessary zinc, B-Complex, and other minerals.

If a nutritional history proves calcium deficiency, then I add calcium supplements. Calcium deficiency was proven to be a cause of reversible cataracts in the early 1950s. With a similar program using only Centrum™, I was successful in improving vision in 67 percent of those patients with cataracts. In some cases vision improved, but the cataract did not appear to change. I have turned my data over to Emory University for their evaluation with a new instrument that can measure changes in the density of the lens, so that we can more precisely determine the effects of various treatments. According to a recent communication from Emory, they have proven that cataracts indeed can be caused by vitamin and mineral deficiencies. In the meantime, I will continue with my shotgun approach to nutritional therapy, which is probably best since isolated deficiencies are rare, and since the various components work together.

Incidentally, since I began using vitamin E in the treatment of cataracts, it has been proven that a vitamin E deficiency will produce reversible cataracts in diabetics.

Senile Macular Degeneration (SMD) is today the number one cause of incurable blindness. The blindness caused by SMD is central, and usually does not destroy side vision. The area affected is only about the size of a human face viewed at conversation distance. Recently, it has been shown that laser therapy, begun soon enough, can be beneficial for about 4 percent of these unfortunate patients. For laser therapy to be effective, the problem must be vascular. If it is vascular, then those vitamins affecting vascular integrity should be effective.

In 1981, while trying to decide how to break the news to a patient with senile macular degeneration, I strongly felt within my spirit that vitamin E and ocean salt would correct her problem. I discussed the disease and treatment options with the lady, who agreed to nutritional therapy. Within six weeks, her vision had improved from 20/60 in each eye to 20/30. Within another six weeks she could see 20/20 in each eye. Since then, I have treated over twenty patients with this disease with very good results: over 90 percent had improved vision. Four patients whose vision had deteriorated to mere hand movement improved sufficiently to read a newspaper (20/50). Please note that improvement may be very slow, taking up to twelve months. Only one patient has had his vision deteriorate while on nutritional treatment, but a few have deteriorated when they stopped the vitamins, only to improve again when therapy was restarted.

It was reported in September, 1983, that the National

Institutes of Health has shown vitamin E to be essential to proper function of the retina, and appears to prevent oxidation of vitamin A. This would appear to confirm my discovery of improved vision in patients with retinal disease when treated with vitamin E.

Dr. Shute had demonstrated that vitamin E, given in sufficient doses, quickly reduces inflammation in diseases such as thrombophlebitis. Since inflammation after cataract surgery is thought to be a main cause for the prolonged recovery time, I decided to use vitamin E post-operatively. Recovery time improved about 50 percent. So I increased the dosage to 1200 IU before and after surgery. Now my patients generally achieve a level of vision within a week that usually took several weeks before. I have had two patients whose vision recovered quickly, then deteriorated with inflammation inside the eye when they discontinued the vitamin without my knowledge. Upon restarting the vitamins their vision returned quickly.

The benefits of vitamin E for treatment of iritis was confirmed by the keynote speaker giving the Jackson Memorial Lecture at the American Academy of Ophthalmology meeting at Chicago on October 31, 1983. It is encouraging that men of such statue are also sufficiently open-minded to overcome past prejudices against nutritional therapy.

I have one patient who has had several bouts of recurrent corneal herpes ulcers, and would not respond to any of the antiviral agents available. During one episode which had lasted several weeks without remission, in desperation I decided to have him instill a drop of vitamin E (which included selenium) in his eye four times daily, and take the rest of the capsule by mouth. Recovery was complete within three days. He has been free of recurrence, using one drop of vitamin E daily, for several years. Previous recurrences were almost every one to two months. His vision is now twice as good as we have been able to obtain anytime within the past several years. A second patient had similar results.

One of the problems I have seen many times is ophthalmic zoster, or shingles. Those unfortunate victims of this disease will attest to the fact that they are miserable, and continue to have severe pain for years after the acute stage is past. Over the years I have developed a procedure of treatment that has been effective in completely preventing pain both during and after the disease, and greatly speeds recovery, with rare exceptions. First, based on Indian studies which have shown prevention of post zoster pain using vitamin B12 injections, I use 1000 micrograms of vitamin B12 injected daily for several days, then weekly thereafter until I am sure they are past the illness. If pain recurs when the dosage of B12 is reduced, it quickly fades when the injections are again increased. It generally takes about three months before the B12 injections can be discontinued altogether. Since the herpes virus has been shown to more readily cause infection when lysine is deficient, I have added lysine either with tablets or with soybean protein. (However, a recent study was not able to confirm that lysine alone would shorten the course of a herpes infection.) Soybean protein is especially rich in lysine. To build up interferon levels, I recommend use of live polio virus to induce rapid production of interferon. It is impossible to sustain two separate viral infections simultaneously. If the patient has ever had live polio virus immunization there is no risk in using live polio virus. The risk is only one in several million for adults who have never been immunized. Injection with Staph phage lysate is also an effective means of boosting interferon levels, and much safer, at least for those who have never been previously immunized against polio. Because inflammation is a severe problem with shingles, I treat with 1200 IU of vitamin E, plus about two grams of vitamin C daily. Finally, I use a potent multivitamin-mineral preparation, plus additional folic acid which must be by prescription. The lesions are generally dry within three days of beginning treatment, if treatment is begun within three days of onset. The victims have no pain, and recover quickly. Even without the interferon boost recovery is remarkably fast.

Recently, a patient came about five days after onset of shingles, and although the protocol was helpful, he was bothered by residual pain. A mutual friend, a physician active in nutritional therapy, suggested intravenous injection of 25 grams of vitamin C. This was done on several occasions, with complete cessation of pain within a few minutes. He was pain free for several hours after each treatment. It took several treatments before he remained pain free. I have no idea how this would work, or if it would be effective in relieving pain in cancer victims, or the composition of the mixture injected. Certainly, this is an area begging for investigation.

Blindness is a major complication of diabetes, and has responded somewhat to laser obliteration of the peripheral retina. It is thought that the disease is due to anoxia, which in turn is due to the poor circulation that diabetics have. The laser therapy is designed to destroy a major portion of the retina so that there will hopefully be sufficient blood left for the remaining retina. It frequently works. Statistically a diabetic with diabetic retinopathy is better off with laser treatment, but the statistics break down when applied to individuals.

There may be a better way. Vitamin E, vitamin C, and bioflavinoids all reduce the need for oxygen. At the same time, they reduce edema from capillary leakage of fluid. These effects should help reduce the anoxia so that new vessels do not develop. Certainly, in diabetic disease of the kidneys this has proven to be the case, and the same process in the kidneys is going on in the eyes.

I encourage all my diabetic patients to go on vitamin C plus bioflavinoids twice daily, 400 IU of vitamin E twice daily, and additionally to take a potent vitamin/mineral preparation. Those who have, have had improved vision, and some mild cases of diabetic retinopathy have cleared completely. More advanced cases probably will still benefit from laser treatment, but I haven't had to refer anyone for laser therapy since beginning intense vitamin therapy about two years ago. Since diabetics cannot convert beta carotenes into vitamin A, they must take vitamin A in addition to consuming foods rich in beta carotenes. They should also take an additional 30 milligrams of zinc, which is available in chelated form. Diabetics also need additional magnesium and manganese. My program is basically what I recommend for almost everyone, except that I encourage those with diabetes to take additional vitamin E, C, and zinc. Refer to the chapter on diabetes for more information.

Too much oxygen is a problem for premature infants, who must have the extra oxygen until their lung tissue develops. Unfortunately, if the amount of oxygen getting into the blood is too great, constriction of small arteries in the peripheral of the eye occurs, followed by scar formation and retinal detachment. In severe cases blindness results. Much research has been done recently, finally confirming that vitamin E, begun within twelve hours of birth, will completely prevent retrolental fibroplasia, the disease form affecting the eyes. Vitamin E does not cross the placental barrier, so every child is born deficient in the vitamin. This deficiency would have been taken care of by the fact that human milk is a good source of vitamin E, assuming the mother is supplementing her diet with the vitamin. Cow's milk is not. Of course, premature infants cannot nurse because they must stay in the incubator. My pediatrician friends assure me that giving vitamin E to premature infants is now standard practice among pediatricians. The reason vitamin E works in apparently opposite conditions is that it acts both as an antioxidant, and by reducing the need of tissues for oxygen.

68

Glaucoma is a disease in which the optic nerve is damaged due to increased pressures within the eye. It is uncertain exactly what actually causes the damage, but it seems to be a combination of restricted blood flow, and restricted flow of fluids within the nerve cells themselves.

The tragedy of glaucoma is that it generally is symptom free until blindness develops. There is, of course, the acute type of glaucoma which can be painful, and is associated with blurred vision. This type is rare, but usually requires immediate surgical treatment by an ophthalmologist. The more common open angle glaucoma is silent. Not only can it cause blindness, but the blindness is of such a nature that the victim seldom will notice it until loss of vision is almost total. It is a difficult situation to explain, but the problem involves the fact that we do not notice something that is not there. A total loss of vision does not appear as black to the victim: it is simply not there. Glaucoma can only be diagnosed and treated by an ophthalmologist, who is a physician with additional training in diseases of the eye. Do not depend on your optometrist to detect glaucoma: the record clearly shows that most do not. They are not physicians and should not be expected to perform a physician's job.

A pressure test is the usual tip-off that glaucoma exists, but the diagnosis depends upon other tests and the expertise of an ophthalmologist. It is a combination of factors, and requires close supervision. Without treatment, blindness is probably inevitable. With treatment, most victims of this disease will enjoy good vision throughout life. Treatment usually consists of use of drops or oral medications. When these fail, as they sometimes do, surgery is usually effective. The worst danger to the glaucoma patient is neglect. Since the disease is inherited, careful examination of all relatives of those with glaucoma is essential. Although glaucoma usually afflicts only those over 30, I have patients with glaucoma who are under eight years of age. Therefore, everyone who is related to a person with glaucoma should be tested. And everyone without a family history should be tested at least by age thirty, although preferably much earlier.

Nutrition may be a factor in some cases of glaucoma. A study done in India this past year demonstrated that patients with glaucoma were usually deficient in vitamin A, as compared to normal persons. Certainly, the incidence of severe vitamin A deficiency in the U.S. is similar to the incidence of glaucoma, and it may also be that persons with a predisposition to glaucoma need more vitamin A. I do have several patients with glaucoma whose pressures dropped to within normal ranges and were able to discontinue medications within a few months of treatment with vitamin A. Since vitamin A requires zinc to be used by the eye, and may also require vitamin E to prevent toxic by-products of vitamin A metabolism, both zinc and vitamin E should be used with vitamin A. I have also had some success treating glaucoma with manganese, 40 milligrams per day. There are some interrelations between vitamin A and manganese that support these results. Since vitamin A deficiencies are slow to reverse, conventional therapy should be begun first, along with vitamin A, vitamin E, zinc and manganese. After about three months, an attempt should be made to discontinue conventional therapy. If not successful, I try again in another three months. The effect of manganese, incidentally, lasts only about two or three days, and may be a pharmocologic effect rather than a benefit of a trace element.

Biotin, taken 1000 micrograms per day, will significantly reduce intraocular pressure in glaucoma patients who apparently are deficient in biotin. The effect occurs within a few days, or it does not occur at all. Glaucoma patients deserve a therapeutic trial of biotin. Manganese is a co-factor within biotin.

Interestingly, some of my patients have not had a notable improvement in pressures, but the appearance of the nerve has markedly improved. This is consistent with our knowledge that glaucoma is a complex disease, and that pressure is not the whole story. Part of the disease is the fact that we vary in our resistance to damage and injury. That difference may in large measure be nutritional in origin.

Warning: since there are no long-term data on nutritional therapy of glaucoma, the patient must be followed at three-month intervals just as though he were under traditional therapy. Also, if vitamin supplementation reverses someone's glaucoma, the glaucoma should be expected to return within time if supplements were discontinued. It may be that those who respond to vitamin therapy are those whose innate need for those vitamins is greater than normal.

Currently, I am testing all of my glaucoma patients for subclinical hypothyroidism; and many, in fact, are hypothyroid. I suspect that abnormal mucopolysaccharides are clogging the drainage holes and that this is reversible.

More recently, Evening primrose oil has been proven in a careful study to reverse diabetic retinopathy. Thyroid hormone has the same effect.

X.
Ulcer Disease

An adequate demonstration of the prevalence of ulcer disease and the pre-ulcer condition of gastric distress is the constant bombardment of antacid advertising on television. The market is certainly there: over twelve million Americans suffer from ulcer disease, fully 5 percent of our population, and over 10 percent of the adult population.

Traditional treatment has been directed at stress management, a totally bland diet, and antacid tablets or liquids. More recently, drugs capable of blocking the production of gastric acid have been introduced, and are remarkably effective. In fact, with these drugs antacid medications are not necessary and do not improve the cure rate. Another effective approach is a medication which totally coats the surface of the stomach, preventing acid from damaging the lining of the stomach. The disadvantage with this approach is that the concoction must be drunk about twenty minutes before each meal, an inconvenience most of us would reject. In addition, I believe that any treatment that works by providing a barrier between food and the stomach and intestines will also block absorption of valuable nutrients.

Although stress has been implicated as a cause of ulcerative disease, it is doubtful that it is a significant factor. Virtually everyone lives under stress, and everyone obviously does not have ulcers. In fact, many with ulcers have very little stress, at least according to their estimation, and likewise many thrive on stress without even the merest hint of an ulcer.

The totally bland Sippy diet used for many years probably is a major source of stress, or at least aggravation at having to eat the stuff, yet there is no statistically valid study proving that a bland diet is effective in either preventing or curing ulcerative disease. In fact, I know of one person with ulcerative problems who says with a straight face that hot peppers are the only thing that will relieve her symptoms. All of us will note a few foods that disagree with our system, and those foods should be avoided. If a spicy food is tasty, and causes no delayed remorse, there is absolutely no reason to miss its pleasure. Alcohol stimulates gastric secretion, a benefit when used with a meal to improve digestion, but certainly a disadvantage when taken on an empty stomach. In my opinion, alcohol has no place except with a meal, and then only in moderation to improve digestion. One of my professors in medical school (before Tagamet™ was available) said that he doubted that the bland diet had any real effect. His experience was that unless the ulcer victim stopped smoking nothing would help, and if they stopped smoking almost anything would be successful.

The most popular bland diet is the Sippy diet for patients with gastric ulcers. One of the main components of the Sippy diet is milk. So why would the Sippy diet have become popular if it were not effective? Perhaps the reason was discovered by Dr. Wilfrid E. Shute, a Canadian physician who spent many decades studying vitamin E and its effects on disease. He had attended a meeting sponsored by Eastman Kodak (a major manufacturer of vitamin E) in which it was pointed out that their scientists could produce ulcers in rats in many ways, but in every case the ulcers would heal promptly with the administration of vitamin E.

About that same time Dr. George Dowd of Worcester, Massachusetts, got interested in the use of vitamin E in treating ulcer disease, and tried it with two patients. One was on a reducing diet, and was not helped. The other was eating a high protein diet (including the milk protein, casein) and was healed promptly. Incidentally, this Dr. Dowd is the first doctor to notice the improvement in eyesight in geriatric patients when they were begun on vitamin E.

A study was then done at Columbia University, demonstrating that rats with ulcers would not heal on vitamin E alone, but healed promptly with the addition of casein (milk protein). Cottage cheese is almost pure casein.

Armed with this information, Dr. Shute discovered that all that was necessary to cure ulcerative disease or gastritis was vitamin E with milk protein in the form of powdered milk. He used 400 IU of vitamin E taken at mid-meal plus three tablespoons of milk powder mixed with water or milk at the end of the meal. Presumedly, vitamin E with cottage cheese or yogurt would also be effective. It is interesting that when the Sippy diet became popular the American diet still supplied a modest amount of vitamin E, far more than now. Another author has found that goat's milk is also effective.

Dr. Shute tells of one man who, against medical advice, used this treatment for a bleeding ulcer, and was well within twenty-four hours. He had already been admitted for surgery but insisted that Dr. Shute's treatment be given a chance first. In addition, Dr. Shute gives two cases in which patients with severe ulcerative colitis responded to large doses of vitamin E.

Certainly, treatment with vitamin E and milk protein is safer and cheaper than any drug available. But don't expect the manufacturer of Tagamet™ to do a study on this approach, since there is no great profit in nutritional therapy. Certainly, milk and vitamin E are beyond patent rights.

Other studies have shown that vitamin A will prevent gastric ulcers in patients under severe stress, the result of burns over a large portion of the body. Whether vitamin A would speed the healing of gastric ulcers has not been studied, to the best of my knowledge. However, the effect of zinc, necessary for the mobilization of vitamin A from stores in the liver, has been studied. In one double-blind study, large doses of zinc given in divided doses resulted in the ulcers healing three times as fast as in the control group. As mentioned elsewhere in this book, copper will also speed the healing of ulcers. Note that vitamin A, zinc, and copper are all involved in DNA and RNA replication, and thus are necessary in any healing process.

Antacid preparations are the mainstay of traditional treatment of ulcers and gastric distress. Virtually all are essentially sodium free, in spite of advertising implying uniqueness of some products. Unfortunately, most of the brands use aluminum compounds as the acid buffer, and aluminum is becoming implicated in several degenerative diseases, including Alzheimer's. Milk of magnesia is an excellent acid buffer that does not contain aluminum, and does contain a useful element (magnesium) although very little of it is absorbed. In excess, various antacid tablets will cause either diarrhea or constipation. In any case, aluminum stimulates free radical production and would be expected to promote degenerative diseases. There is increasing evidence that aluminum toxicity is a major cause of Alzheimer's, Parkinson's Disease, loss of memory and premature aging. I personally believe the evidence is strong enough that I will not knowingly consume products made with aluminum (such as antacids), nor cooked for prolonged periods in aluminum vessels (unless coated with Teflon). I don't see a problem with aluminum foil. However, the amount of aluminum picked up by beverages in aluminum cans needs to be examined very carefully. Aluminum salts are a major ingredient in self-rising flours, baking powder, and many food mixes. Read the label and avoid those products. Aluminum salts are also the active ingredient in most anti-perspirant preparations, and act after being absorbed through the skin. We may have to accept a world that is a little less "sanitary" and convenient as the price for better health. The jury is still out on this one. In any case, chelation will remove aluminum ions from the body.

However, the advantages of the various antacid preparations is hardly worth the discussion, because there is absolutely no evidence that they are of any benefit in curing gastric or duodenal ulcers. They do give temporary relief to the pain of an ulcer, but a glass of milk will do as much. If Dr. Shute is correct, then that glass of milk, plus vitamin E, may be a lot more effective.

There are two other treatments for ulcer disease claimed to be effective. For stomach ulcers, it is said that the juice of a fresh Irish potato, drunk *immediately* after it is extracted with a juicer, is curative. For duodenal ulcers, the mixture of potato juice and cabbage juice (apparently a fairly foul tasting mixture) is claimed to be effective. In both cases, the juice must be prepared fresh and consumed immediately. This is interesting, since fresh potato juice *is* effective in relieving the pain of solar keratitis (burns on the corneas (eyes) of welders, or those overexposed to ultraviolet light). Coenzyme Q10 has also been proven to speed recovery from ulcer disease.

Copper and zinc are essential for healing, and patients with ulcer disease (both of skin and the digestive tract) are frequently deficient in one or both elements. For example, aspirin is known to produce gastric ulcers. Aspirin chelates copper in the walls of the stomach and removes it to the site of inflammation. This leaves a deficiency in the stomach, which prevents normal healing from occurring. Copper salicylate (aspirin) will not only not cause ulcers, it will heal gastric ulcers.

Treating ulcer disease is not part of my specialty, but I would be very interested in getting input from any patient or physician who tries one of these methods, either successfully or otherwise. Good luck!

Postscript: I have now had several persons write of success using the milk and Vitamin E approach. One had been using Tagamet™ for six months, and was free of pain within a week! One person has written and claimed success with cabbage juice. All who have written noted prompt recovery.

XI.
In Case of Nuclear Accident

Most of us have visions of Hiroshima and the end of the world when we think of a nuclear accident. Certainly, with the proliferation of nuclear weapons, and especially of nuclear weapon technology, a nuclear war or accident is entirely possible. I rather doubt that the United States, Great Britain, or France would be first to push the nuclear button. I also doubt that either India or China would be willing to use their weapons, but I believe China is more to be trusted in this regard. It is the Soviet Union we should fear most, because they have demonstrated time and again that they are willing to sacrifice innocent lives to win their objectives if there is a good possibility of winning. Further, the Soviet Union covertly finances and promotes worldwide terrorism as a tool for disrupting free societies and eventual conquest. Eventually, unless international terrorism is stopped, some group will turn to nuclear technology as the ultimate terrorist tool.

The most likely nuclear accident will be from sabotage or malfunction of a nuclear power plant, and even this risk is extremely small. So far, there have been no deaths or injuries due to the operation of nuclear power plants, a safety record no other energy source can approach. The claim that there is no way to dispose of nuclear wastes is unfounded. There are at least two methods of safely processing and disposing of nuclear wastes, one of which has been used in Europe for over five years. The tremendous pileup of nuclear wastes in this country is due to political timidity in the face of fanatic militant ignorance.

A nuclear accident can produce four different types of radiation. Alpha radiation consists of high-speed, heavy, positively-charged particles identical to the nucleus of a helium atom. Alpha particles cannot penetrate the skin. However, if an alpha particle emitter is ingested it can produce a lot of damage internally. Fallout from a nuclear accident (or war) will produce a lot of alpha radiation. Protection from alpha radiation consists of having a clean water supply (distillation would be effective) and keeping fallout dust from any foods. Cleanliness will definitely be next to godliness after a nuclear accident.

Beta radiation consists of a high-speed electron ejected from an atom during nuclear decay. Again, beta radiation does not penetrate deeply, but would be most dangerous if ingested. Even a thin shelter would protect against beta radiation.

Gamma radiation consists of high energy electromagnetic waves emitted at the instant of nuclear detonation. As with all radiation, gamma radiation produces its damage by production of free radicals. Like X-rays, gamma rays penetrate deeply, and requires a thick shield of earth, concrete, or lead to block their damage. On the positive side, intense gamma radiation will persist only for a few days after a nuclear accident. If a gamma source is ingested, it will produce its damage internally. But a gamma source is just as dangerous when it is close outside the body.

Neutron radiation will occur only for a brief instant upon the detonation of a nuclear device. A nuclear device can be designed to produce mainly neutron radiation. There is virtually no way to shield against neutron radiation, and once the blast is over there is minimal residual radiation. The damage produced is due to the instantaneous production of billions of free radicals.

However, those who would ban nuclear power plants because of the radiation emitted are ignorant. Coal contains natural radioactive particles, which are released with fly ash when coal is burned. In fact, your exposure to radiation as a result of coal-burning electric facilities far exceeds what you would get if all electricity were generated from nuclear power. I am not in favor of nuclear fission reactors, however, because I believe that type of power should be reserved for those uses in which there is no alternative: nuclear-powered ships, submarines, and spacecraft. Safer sources of energy are solar, wind (a form of solar power), and nuclear fusion. Renewable energy sources such as alcohol and wood need to be used, but wood, especially, is producing significant pollution already, while destroying the planet's ability to deal with pollution. Small hydroelectric power plants can also contribute significantly to our renewable energy supply. Dollar for dollar, the cheapest source is conservation. Energy efficient machines and homes will allow us to maintain our standard of living without exhausting our energy sources.

Still, we have a problem, and must deal with it. *All* radiation produces damage by the formation of free radicals, the same free radicals that are formed by smog, peroxidized fats, and metal ions including aluminum, cadmium, copper, and iron. The damage you would sustain while sleeping in a nuclear power plant during a coolant leak is far less than the free radical damage sustained from smoking one cigarette, or eating fries at the local fast food restaurant. In fact, since cosmic radiation is identical to gamma radiation, you would sustain more damage flying across the nation in a jet aircraft, or sunbathing a few hours on the beach. So let's get things into their proper perspective. It is the free radicals that are killing us, and nuclear radiation is merely one possible source of free radicals. It is tragic to see our citizens marching in protest against a nuclear power plant, smoking their cigarettes (or whatever), and eating their free radical-producing fast food lunches, when the alternative is many times more dangerous than nuclear power. If you are sincerely against nuclear power, then adjust your lifestyle to minimal energy usage so that we will not be forced into building nuclear power plants, or running our dangerous fossil fuel plants at full capacity. The improvement in technology is such that within two decades viable alternate choices will be readily available.

Combating free radical damage will be discussed fully in a later chapter. The main thing to know at this point is that radiation damage is due to free radicals, and is absolutely no different than free radical damage from the foods we eat, or the smog we inhale.

Radioactive iodine, a major isotope in radioactive fallout, is most dangerous if ingested because iodine is selectively taken up by the thyroid gland. If the iodine taken up is radioactive and of sufficient quantity it can destroy the thyroid gland. In fact, this is used therapeutically in some cases of hyperthyroidism. In lower doses, there is an increased risk of thyroid cancer. If you already have sufficient iodine in your system, there will be no additional iodine taken up, whether radioactive or not. By having your physician write you a prescription of supersaturated potassium iodide, 30cc per person, and taking it immediately when a nuclear accident appears imminent you can prevent damage from radioactive iodine. The proper immediate dose would be about six drops in a glass of water, repeated three times a day for about two weeks. Since our diet already supplies many times the minimum amount of iodine needed, there is no need to take additional supplemental iodine on a regular basis. There is no harm unless you are allergic to iodine. This would saturate your thyroid gland with non-radioactive iodine and prevent any significant amount of radioactive iodine from being absorbed.

Radioactive strontium will be selectively taken up by bone,

and was a real problem for several years after we discontinued atmospheric nuclear testing. Radioactive strontium fallout in pastureland was eaten by cattle, and showed up in their milk. Since calcium and strontium compete with each other, taking a generous calcium supplement will not only help prevent strontium uptake by your bones, but will remove strontium already deposited there. It may turn out that strontium is an essential trace element, in which case supplemental strontium would also be indicated.

Plutonium and other heavy metals also are toxic (extremely so) when ingested. Vitamin C, several grams a day, and chelation will effectively remove these elements.

I do not believe that a nuclear war is inevitable. Nor do I believe that a nuclear freeze will prevent war. The only rational defense is to make potential aggressors think twice before going to war, and that means that we of the free world must develop whatever means necessary to defend ourselves, and to inflict unacceptable damage on our enemies. For this reason I am strongly in favor of space defense weapons, and of deploying neutron weapons which will not cause a "nuclear winter." Such weapons will give any potential aggressor ample cause to pause before going to war. Rewarding aggression will only encourage further aggression. Unfortunately, the cost of freedom is eternal vigilance, for which we must pay the price.

The next few decades are critical for the human race, and for Earth itself. So get informed and get involved. Do not leave the final decisions to politicians or radical groups who do not have your interests at heart.

Note: The 1986 Chernobyl reactor accident clearly demonstrated that nuclear accidents are possible. The devastation is such that it appears to have cooled the Soviet's taste for war. Of greater interest, read Revelation 8:10-11 (in the Bible): the falling star means a city is destroyed. Chernobyl is the Ukrainian word for "wormwood." A coincidence? You decide.

XII.
Age Is More Than Years

For most of my life I have been told that our life is but threescore and ten, or by virtue of good health perhaps fourscore. In medical school, we were taught that during Roman times life expectancy was only thirty-five years, and that the improvement today is the result of medical science.

Both of these assumptions are false. Were the life expectancy of Roman citizens a mere thirty-five years, their civilization would never have developed because no one would have lived long enough to pass the elements of their culture along to the next generation. Continuity of culture must exist for civilization to develop. A brief reading of Greek and Roman history will assure you that many of that day lived past ninety. Socrates was over ninety when the state made him commit suicide for corrupting the youth by teaching them that there was only one God. Obviously, they felt they could not wait for a natural death, so Socrates must have been in good health at the time.

As an aside, the past two decades in the United States of America have seen a deliberate, and successful, attempt by the humanists to prevent the teaching of the current younger genera-tion the values that have made our civilization great. We are witnessing the remaking of a great civilization into an alien image. Our American civilization, the greatest the world has ever known, was built by men inspired by the Holy Scriptures of its Jewish and Christian immigrants. America is the direct result of scriptural influence: men who know that they are sons of God will bow to no man nor government. They are free. To prevent that influence from being passed on to the next generation is cultural genocide. This is an aside, but one worthy of your thought.

The "threescore and ten" comes from the Bible, but is not a statement of how long we should live, but how long most lived in those days. David, who wrote those verses, lived to age 70. Actually, there is a promise in Scripture that sets a limit on lifespan, but that limit is 120 years (Genesis 6:3). There is also a promise that the day will come when anyone who lives less than a hundred years will be as one cut off early, and those who live a life in harmony with the Spirit of God will live the long life of a tree (Isaiah 65: 20-22). The promise is a life of many hundreds of years for those who are walking in harmony with the Creator. I believe this generation will see this prophecy fulfilled.

This limit is very interesting, because within the decade it has been discovered that the human genetic code has a genetic clock that appears to be timed to shut us down at about 120 years. The way I understand it, the clock allows a limited number of repairs of major cell systems, so that when these cells have reproduced the set number of times they will no longer reproduce. Within a few weeks of that event the body will age precipitously and die. This is consistent with our clinical experience, for we all know of persons who seemed not to age, but in old age (usually about 90 to 100) they suddenly deteriorated and died within a very few weeks. I believe their genetic clock had shut them down.

The existence of this clock has some interesting philosophical and practical implications. First, since the clock actually counts repair cycles, we obviously shorten our lives with each major (and minor?) illness, and with each time we allow ourselves to deteriorate physically by lack of exercise or poor nutrition. The elimination of childhood diseases may have had a major effect on longevity other than simply allowing more people to live longer. From a practical point, then, we might be able to lengthen our lives simply by being consistent in good health practices: exercise, good nutrition, and adequate rest.

To me, the philosophical implications are even more interesting. If there is a limit on lifespan, then our Creator has no intention of letting us live forever in this body, just as a caterpillar must die so that the butterfly can emerge. Indeed, current studies in life after death have fairly solidly shown that our conscious life is in no way limited by this physical body. From the standpoint of this life, if there had to be a limit on lifespan, then aging itself is a disease, and should not occur under ideal conditions. That is to say, if aging were a normal sequence of events, then death would follow automatically, and there would be no need to put a limit on lifespan. Just as there are persons who age abnormally fast, there are those who do not appear to age until shortly before death, giving weight to this hypothesis.

Certainly, the human brain is capable of learning from more experience than can be had in even centuries of life, even life lived to the fullest. The excess mental capacity of the human brain is staggering. The recent invention of CT scanning (a modern medical miracle) has uncovered the astounding fact that there are some persons, fully normal in intellect and abilities, who are achieving this with a mere 5 percent of their brain intact! The rest of their brain had been destroyed by hydrocephalus which had been surgically arrested in infancy. Although these persons were outwardly normal, most of their brain had been destroyed. In fact, some of these persons are professional and have achieved academic honors. This is in line with the conclusions of a team of neurosurgeons, who concluded that the center of intelligence and personality is not the brain. They concluded that man is a creature that uses machines, and the body and brain are merely two of the machines he uses. In short, our limitations are those we impose upon ourselves.

I am suggesting that if we could discover the factors which lead to optimum health, we would discover that aging would not occur until shortly before death. We would live a vigorous life, perpetually young, through perhaps the age of 120 years, then age suddenly and die swiftly and easily. Not a bad life, and not a bad way to go.

Is this a reasonable expectation? Nutrition and aging research with animals has clearly demonstrated that life extension on the order of 30 to 50 percent is easily possible. More interesting for the theory I am proposing is the fact that these animals continue to have the behavior typical of young animals until shortly before death. Three decades ago most American pets were fed table scraps, and an old dog survived to perhaps twelve years. Today, most dogs are fed scientifically designed food and many live as many as eighteen years. Good nutrition has added 50 percent to their life span. If such a simple measure as good nutrition has increased their lifespan by 50 percent, it seems reasonable that humans could live to 120 years by using the same approach.

Other animal studies have shown that animals deprived of calories, but abundantly fed vitamins and minerals, also maintain their youth far beyond the useful lifespan. Just cutting calories won't work; it must be a low calorie, high nutrition diet. Dr. Roy Walford, a professor of pathology at UCLA, is testing these concepts on himself. I believe he will be successful: the evidence in animal studies is almost overwhelming.

About a decade ago, NASA funded research on aging, because travel to the stars will take thousands of years with today's technology, and obviously is impossible unless aging can be prevented. One of the discoveries made was that the elderly can tolerate exercise and stress just as well as young persons. One conclusion was that we grow old because we are too lazy not to. That is very true. Most of us are too lazy to put out the effort and bear the discomfort necessary to maintain our physical strength and health. Most of us are surviving in a slowly deteriorating body which complains with aches and pains when we do anything out of the ordinary, hoping we will live out our threescore and ten and die an easy death. When we do exert ourselves, we discover places where we didn't know we had places, and attribute this to old age. Then we vow not to try that again, and continue the inevitable slide toward the grave. When we were younger, we would have gotten sore just as now, but would have correctly attributed the soreness to being out of shape, and would have pushed harder to whip ourselves into some semblance of human form. We have aged because our attitudes about aging have allowed us to deteriorate: we have lowered our standards and accepted less than optimal health as the best that we could achieve, then fell short in even that modest goal. We have become prisoners within our own bodies. The ultimate irony is that we are also the prison wardens.

I have watched with sadness as older citizens age and give up trying, justifying their actions by their self-imposed limits of threescore and ten. As they reach their mid-60s, they begin to slow down and prepare to die. And then they do exactly what they have been saying that they would do, dying at the magic number of threescore and ten. This is no different than an African native who is killed by a hex by the local witch doctor: they believe they are going to die, and they die. I recently visited some older friends who are now in their late 60s. Their automobile and home is in need of repair, and they can afford the expense. But, they justify their not bothering by saying that there is no need to buy a new car when they will be here for so short a time. Yet, they are still vigorous and active, nowhere near death were it not for their negative attitude. Unless someone is able to break their attitude of impending death they will die decades prematurely. If a negative attitude can shorten life, and it can, then a positive attitude can prolong the length of days, or at least sustain that which we have. Obviously, we cannot by positive thought cheat death, but we can prevent death from visiting earlier than necessary. So set down and adjust your attitude and then start taking the steps necessary to live life to its fullest.

There are five factors which affect lifespan. First, you should be careful in selecting your parents, since good genetic material lends itself to a long life. Obviously, this you cannot control.

However, if you are fortunate enough to have a strong ancestry, be kind enough to the human race to more than reproduce your kind. If you have severe genetic weaknesses, then do the race a favor and limit your progeny.

Second, take time to exercise and use your body, pushing it daily to beyond your previous limits. It is true in every field of life: if you don't use it, you lose it. Deterioration due to lack of exercise starts almost immediately, as proven by even the short orbital space flights. However, from a practical point, exercise indulged in at least three times weekly can maintain whatever status you have attained. Moderate exercise is best, and the exercise should occupy at least a half-hour daily. Moderate exercise such as walking is more likely to be continued throughout life, and therefore be more useful than jogging which is too strenuous for many, and may therefore not be done consistently. Daily, regular, moderate exercise is the key. Riding a golf cart each weekend simply doesn't hack it. If moderate exercise leaves you sore, get serious while you still have a body that can get sore, and try to recover your loss by a slow and progressive exercise program. Many such programs have been designed and are readily available. Plan for the long haul: your exercise program will last you a lifetime, and will either prolong or foreshorten that day. So plan a program you can live with, make it daily, make it long, and make it hard enough to raise a sweat. In research done by Dr. Kenneth Cooper on conditioning, he concluded that at least twelve minutes of vigorous activity, done at least three times weekly, is necessary to produce cardiac conditioning. If you jog, use special shoes with Sorbothane™ to reduce the risk of damage to your knees and ankles, or use a jogging trampoline.

Incidentally, strenuous exercise will *not* substitute for nutritional supplements or judicious use of chelation therapy. Exercise will enlarge critical arteries, and reduce the risk of premature death, but will not reverse or prevent atherosclerosis or other free radical pathology, although there will be some benefit in that direction.

Third is attitude, which was discussed above. If you believe aging is natural and inevitable, you will not look for ways to avoid it. Not that you should get depressed with aging changes, now that you no longer look like a teenager. Full maturity is reached in the late 20s or early 30s, not at age 18. Your goal should be to maintain the vigor of that maturity, not the foolishness of youth.

Fourth, you must eliminate from your life those toxic substances which can be avoided. Along with these toxic substances I would include stressful environments and people. Stay away from people and things that are bad for you. Foremost among these is tobacco in all its forms, including secondhand smoke. If possible, avoid chlorinated water by using well water, or by a special filter designed to remove chlorine. Chlorine can also be removed by boiling the water, or simply letting it stand overnight in an open container. You can protect yourself against environmental pollution by increasing your intake of the antioxidant vitamins and minerals, especially the beta carotenes, B-complex, C, E, zinc, and selenium. There is increasing evidence that foods containing caffeine are toxic. As with most things, your body can handle almost anything in moderation. The evidence concerning alcohol is mixed. In moderation, alcoholic beverages appear to be beneficial, especially the wines and beers. Indeed, it is said that the human body produces the equivalent of two quarts of beer daily. Distilled spirits have no redeeming virtues to recommend them, except as an automotive fuel. Used to intoxication, there is no question that alcohol does permanent damage, and can shorten your life quickly when combined with strong emotions or with driving. If you cannot drink without getting drunk, don't drink at all. This is one area where moderation is a real virtue. And, of course, alcohol affects performance at far lower levels than legally allowed for driving. The wise man will not drink before driving. Nor will a wise woman drink if there is any possibility whatsoever that she might be pregnant.

Fifth, the nutritional approaches to longevity are generally the same as those proposed to fight cancer, since both are the result of oxidation. Good nutrition should begin with prenatal nutrition, and continue throughout life. It is especially important during the growing years from birth through age 20, since defects due to poor nutrition produced during growth will never be fully overcome. In fact, free radical damage inflicted on an unborn child by poor nutrition will affect the child's health for his entire life. Longevity is best promoted by a childhood diet that is rich in vitamins and minerals, but limited in calories and restricted in fat and protein. Sugar and refined flour products are too toxic to allow in the diet of any child. Enough protein is essential, of course, but too much protein seems to promote aging. Perhaps this is the result of free radical formation accompanying the ingestion of fats and iron associated with animal proteins. A good argument can be made that the accelerated aging associated with a high protein diet is due to the fat and iron taken along with most protein sources. In any case, the optimum amount of protein to be included in the diet is yet to be determined.

Especially important in childhood is the restriction of white sugar and flour. I would recommend total avoidance of both. Don't even let your child know there is such a thing as sweets for as long as possible. Animals which are never allowed to taste sweets will naturally select nutritious foods when given a choice. Once white sugar is introduced to the diet, they seem to lose that ability to choose wisely. They go for the sweet foods and ignore the highly nutritious. Sugar is distinctly addicting, and further promotes the overgrowth of Candida albicans, the source of many food allergies and toxic reactions.

The average American gets most of his calories from fat, with processed sugar being the second source of calories. Except for a few essential fats, both are devoid of nutritional value, and deplete the body of essential vitamins and minerals. My recommendation would be to limit calories from fat to perhaps 25 percent of the total. This is merely 500 calories, or 55 grams of fat, found in just under two ounces daily. I believe the safest form of fat to be butter, or fresh vegetable oils. If you do use vegetable oils, be sure they are fresh and increase your intake of the antioxidant vitamins. One way of getting high-quality protein without extra fat calories is to eat more seafoods, or poultry (without the skins), or substitute soybean protein to which methionine has been added. If you do this, you can reduce the daily requirement for protein to about 45 grams. (See Chapter 26 for more on fats.)

Fill out your diet with fresh fruit and vegetables, preferably eaten raw from your own garden. Insofar as possible, try to develop a small organic garden site to grow much of your food. It may take years to restore the soil to full health, but the rewards will be well worth it. A small garden is not only a source of nutrition, but exercise, and relaxation. A garden is excellent therapy for the stresses of modern living.

I would like to recommend the book *Life Extension* for your study, although I believe their solutions are too extreme to be practical. They have documented the growing amount of scientific evidence pointing to a longer, healthier life. I believe the principles they mention are valid, and can be achieved at a cost less than the cost of a pack of cigarettes a day. Good health will repay the modest cost by reduced health care costs, and increased productivity.

As far as actual supplementation, I would recommend a modest program including those supplements listed in a later chapter. I believe this to be a practical approach to better health, and not extravagant nor deficient. Following these suggestions may not prolong your life to the Biblical promise of 120 years, but will make those you live more enjoyable and productive.

In view of the increasingly polluted nature of ground water and city water supplies, the family seriously interested in their health should carefully consider purchasing a home distillery unit capable of producing 3-12 gallons of distilled water per day. Since units cost approximately $1000, one should have a careful analysis of his water performed first to see whether the expense is worth while. However, if your water has a bad taste, or leaves stains in your sinks or bathtubs, a water distillery is very much worth considering.

Distilled water not only operates more efficiently in the body, it does not bring with it the pollutants of modern society. Chlorine, especially, has been proven to produce atherosclerosis in animals, and very probably has the same effect in man. In any case, chlorine does neutralize vitamin E, and the benefits of vitamin E are well known.

Although controversial, use of 1 to 4 drops of 35% *food grade* hydrogen peroxide per glass of water seems to be beneficial. Users claim it works by boosting tissue oxygen levels. I believe it works by causing the body to produce extra superoxide dismutase (SOD). If you elect to try hydrogen peroxide, use only food grade products, and begin at a low dose of one or two drops daily.

Unprocessed fruit, rain and spring water, and raw vegetables also supply hydrogen peroxide, which may explain their benefits.

Coenzyme Q10, recently available at modest cost, has been proven to prolong life, slow the aging process, and appears to actually reverse aging. It is naturally present in organ meats (heart, liver, kidney, pancreas) and it is totally non-toxic. A reasonable dose would be 30 to 300 milligrams per day, for a total of about 3000 milligrams over one to three months. A reasonable maintenance dose would be 30 milligrams per day. If you see no benefit after about 1000 milligrams you are probably not deficient. It is proven effective for reducing blood pressure, obesity, and sugar levels in diabetics.

XIII.
Cholesterol:
A Mixed Blessing

If you are approaching middle age, and are not yet concerned about cholesterol, you have a marvelous ability to ignore a constant bombardment from television ads, radio, your friends, and your physician. You are being advised to stop eating saturated fats (beef, butter, lard), and switch to unsaturated vegetable fats and margarine. You have been advised to stop eating eggs, which contain a lot of cholesterol, and get your nutrition as best you can.

You have been given bad advice.

Cholesterol is a compound manufactured within your body to meet certain needs of the body. Cholesterol is so important that virtually every cell in the body produces it. It is the starting point for producing hormones, vitamin D, and bile. Without cholesterol, you cannot grow, you cannot digest your food, you will not mature, and you will die. Although the average American diet, rich in cholesterol, supplies about 500 milligrams of cholesterol, your body will synthesize an additional 2000 milligrams daily. If you eat more, you will synthesize less. If you eat less, you will synthesize more. Totally eliminating cholesterol from your diet will not materially affect your blood cholesterol levels. Each egg you eat contains about 250 milligrams of cholesterol, and helps your body by eliminating the need for you to synthesize that amount. You could eat as many as six eggs daily without affecting your blood cholesterol levels, if they were properly cooked. So, include up to perhaps two eggs in your daily diet. You need the good nutrition eggs provide. Those foods which are good sources of cholesterol are also very nutritious.

Still, a high blood level of LDL cholesterol (the toxic form) is clearly associated with cardio-vascular disease. If diet does not affect the level of cholesterol in the blood, what will?

It turns out that there are basically two types of cholesterol, a reduced wholesome form, and a toxic peroxidized form. The reduced (good) form attaches itself to a high-density lipoprotein (HDL). The toxic peroxidized form is associated with a low-density lipoprotein (LDL), and is excreted via bile if there is enough vitamin C in the diet. In its natural form, egg yolk is a rich source of the good reduced form of cholesterol, and is both wholesome and beneficial. If the yolk membrane is broken during cooking, or used in a batter mixture, the cholesterol quickly oxidizes to the toxic form. That is why eggs boiled, poached, or cooked sunny side up are wholesome, but cooked scrambled, or in an omelet, or pastry are harmful.

About two decades ago, a study was done in which a group of middle-aged men, all with high blood cholesterol levels, were divided into two groups. One group was put on a low cholesterol diet, the second group was put on a high cholesterol diet. Each group was then further divided into two groups each. One group was allowed to continue as before, the second group was put on an ever-increasing exercise regimen which led to their jogging about a mile daily by the end of the study. The cholesterol levels of those who did not enter into an exercise program remained high: diet had no significant effect on cholesterol levels. Of those who were exercising vigorously, cholesterol levels dropped significantly; again, diet had no real effect. The conclusion is obvious: dietary cholesterol (if in its beneficial reduced form), within reason, will not affect blood cholesterol levels. Even moderate exercise will. Even more significantly, exercise increases the high-density lipid levels while decreasing the low-density lipid levels. This shift is very good.

High blood cholesterol levels could be due to any one of three factors: too much produced, to much ingested, or too little removed from the body. The experiment with exercise clearly shows us that the amount we ingest is of no consequence: the problem lies with over-production, or with poor elimination. Both have proven to be important factors.

Elevated cholesterol levels may also indicate hypothyroidism, highly likely since perhaps 40 percent of our population is hypothyroid. I urge you to read Dr. Langer's book (see reading list) for a thorough discussion of this largely ignored disease.

Cholesterol is a potent antioxidant, scavenging free radicals from our bodies, those highly charged molecules which can produce cellular damage, leading to aging and/or cancer. Cholesterol is one of our natural defense mechanisms against this enemy. But only one defense. It should be noted at this point that fat in the diet is a major source of both free radicals and cholesterol, therefore calories supplied by fat should be reduced to 25 percent, a significant reduction for most of us. Other defenses include vitamin A, beta carotene, vitamin B-1 (Thiamine), vitamin B-3 (Niacin), vitamin B-5 (pantothenic acid), vitamin B-6 (Pyridoxine), vitamin C, vitamin E, chromium, manganese, silicon, selenium, vanadium, and zinc. Copper and iron are beneficial, but only if there is not an excess. Of these, the only one we can produce within the body is cholesterol; the rest must be part of our diet. Provide the proper nutrients, and your body will not have to manufacture so much cholesterol to defend itself against a hostile environment.

It turns out that the advice to stop eating eggs, and to substitute unsaturated oils for saturated fats such as butter has been a serious mistake. First, in eliminating eggs we eliminated excellent nutrition without reducing the cholesterol levels one iota. In addition, we forced the body to use precious resources to produce the extra cholesterol needed.

Second, in substituting unsaturated oils for butter and shortening, we substituted a product that is *much* more susceptible to oxidation than the saturated fats. The oxidation of fats produces the very toxic products we should be trying to avoid: namely, the free radicals. Rancid oils are probably the most common source of carcinogens, other than tobacco products, that we are apt to use daily. In our effort to reduce cholesterol, we have increased the body's need for it.

L-Carnitine, taken 250 milligrams twice daily, will reduce blood cholesterol levels within two weeks. L-Carnitine is more effective taken with essential fatty acids or Evening primrose oil. Carnitine is a vitamin-like substance found in meat.

Bioflavinoids, especially quercitin, are very effective in reducing blood cholesterol. They are especially effective along with L-Carnitine and essential fatty acids in reducing blood triglycerides.

Six months ago, I decided to abandon my generally low cholesterol diet, and switch from margarine to butter. I also switched to the antioxidant supplement discussed in this chapter. As a result, my cholesterol dropped from 289 to 189, in spite of a weight gain and general lack of exercise during that period of time. By increasing my exercise levels and decreasing my weight, I will improve that figure even more.

Fiber is another means of controlling cholesterol. Toxic peroxidized cholesterol is excreted into the small intestine along with bile which helps in the absorption of fats and fat soluble vitamins. A high fiber diet will trap a good bit of that cholesterol in the intestine so that it is removed from the body. And incidentally, additional vitamin C and choline will make the cholesterol more soluble so that gallstones are less likely to be formed. Cholesterol gallstones can also be dissolved using increased quantities of vitamin C and choline. Choline is essential to mobilize and dissolve plaques of cholesterol from blood vessels.

In summary, if you have a high cholesterol problem, the problem is not one of too much in the diet. The problem may be one of too many free radicals combined with too little physical activity. It may also be due to hypothyroidism, the best test for which is the basal temperature test. If your resting oral temperature is below 97.8 you are hypothyroid, and treatment is indicated. The cure is fivefold: first, work with your physician and set up a gradually increasing program of daily exercise. This is extremely important: not only does it reduce cholesterol and increase the HDL fraction, but exercise is a potent tranquillizer, and stress is known to elevate cholesterol levels. Second, take choline liberally to dissolve the cholesterol deposits from your arteries and mobilize so that it may be excreted. Third, increase your vitamin C intake to keep the cholesterol soluble and thereby avoid gallstones during the cleansing period. Vitamin C will also reduce your need to keep the cholesterol levels high. As little as 250 milligrams daily is effective, but if you are serious about a cholesterol problem take at least a gram daily. Initially, vitamin C will increase blood cholesterol levels as cholesterol deposits are dissolved. Fourth, increase your intake of the other anti-oxidant nutrients. And, finally, increase your fiber intake. Natural fiber is an excellent source of silicon, and also tends to trap the excreted toxic cholesterol so that it is not resorbed. Not all fiber is effective, however, but only those natural fibers which contain minerals and perhaps unknown factors. Niacin, 50 to 300 milligrams (will cause a strong hot flush), taken several times per day, will drastically drop cholesterol levels. One should begin with low levels and gradually increase to tolerance. This is more effective with vitamin E, C, and lecithin. Coenzyme 10 and N,N Dimethylglycine have also been proven to reduce cholesterol levels. Both are natural food products and are totally non-toxic.

Many of these needs can be met by switching your diet away from animal proteins toward a vegetarian diet. I do not advocate a complete vegetarian diet, although that can be very healthy when done properly. What I am suggesting is to make vegetables the main part of your meal, rather than follow the usual American practice of making meat the main course, with vegetables merely an after-thought. The pure vegetarian diet is usually deficient in vitamin B-12, and in some amino acids. The simplest solution is to eat some animal protein daily. Remember that vitamin B12 must come from meat, or from a supplement.

Cholesterol is a blessing involved in the vital functions of every cell. It becomes a curse when environmental pollution, poor diet, and lazy health habits force the body to over produce cholesterol for its own protection. The solution is not to eliminate cholesterol from the diet, but to eliminate the causes for its excess. Our approach to cholesterol should be a classic example of not throwing the baby out with the bath water. High cholesterol is not a disease, it is the result of major insults to our bodies through a lack of physical activity and proper diet. The holistic approach I have described will work, and is cheaper and safer than any drug on the market. I challenge you to put this approach to good use in your life.

XIV.
The Natural Prevention of Cancer

I need to state from the outset that I do not have any magic cure for cancer, nor am I soliciting cancer patients. However, experience teaches us that the best cure is prevention, and in that sense there is a natural cure for cancer. Hopefully, someday we will be able to confirm that the prevention is also a cure, or at least an adjunct to other therapy. Read on for some very enlightening details.

About 20 percent of deaths today are due to cancer, so that we can say that of the 240 million Americans alive today, 48 million will probably die of cancer. Even more important, according to the National Academy of Sciences report on Diet, Nutrition, and Cancer (1982), 30 to 40 percent of cancers in men, and 60 percent of cancers in women, are due to diet. Smoking accounts for another 50 percent of cancer in men, and is an increasing factor in women. Taken together, diet and smoking cause fully 90 percent of all deaths due to cancer. Translated into other terms, if all use of tobacco were eliminated and proper diet were followed over 43 million Americans now alive would not die of cancer. If you like to think in financial terms, this wasting of human life will cost us over a trillion health care dollars over the next few decades.

Although there is much more to be learned in the field of nutrition and its relationship to disease, the academy was able to make some interim guideline suggestions.

First, there is sufficient evidence that the consumption of fat is linked with many common cancers. More specifically, it is the oxidized fats and fats altered by processing or hydrogenation which are the problem. Fatty acids, including essential fatty acids, are incorporated into cell walls (membranes). If those fatty acids have been altered by processing, they are still incorporated into the cell membrane, but do not function normally. The cell membrane is not just a piece of material like a sheet of plastic, it is a functional part of the cell, and has very important tasks to perform. Among those tasks is to keep vital ions inside the cell, and other ions out. A healthy cell membrane actively pumps potassium and magnesium into the cell, and calcium and sodium out. When a muscle contracts, or a nerve transmits an impulse, there is a partial reversal of these ions, which must be repositioned by the pump mechanism. A faulty cell membrane is leaky, and leaks calcium and sodium into the cell, and results in the loss of intracellular ions such as potassium, chromium, selenium, and magnesium. Unsaturated fats, the vegetable oils and products so highly advertised, are easily oxidized by exposure to air (both during processing and consumption), producing lipid peroxides (free radicals) which are highly toxic. It would therefore be prudent to curtail our intake of fat by whatever means. Most easily would be to shift from fried to boiled, steamed, or broiled foods, and to choose vegetable sources of protein (which contain less fat) over animal proteins. A reduction in fat consumption by as much as 25 percent is expected to produce meaningful benefits. (The average American diet provides 45 percent of its calories from fat. This should be reduced to about 25 percent.)

Second, our diets should be shifted toward more fruit, vegetables, and whole grain cereals. The cruciferous vegetables (cabbage, broccoli, cauliflower, and brussels sprouts) seem to be especially effective in suppressing the formation of cancer at various sites. Other apparently beneficial nutrients are the beta carotenes which produce the yellow color in many fruit and vegetables. Beta carotenes are also richly found in dark green vegetables, especially broccoli. However, it is the eating of wholesome food that confers the benefits: supplements of individual nutrients have not been shown to be effective. Yet.

Third, smoked and salt cured foods increase the risk of cancer, and their use should be minimized.

Fourth, food additives pose a risk of cancer, and should be used only where necessary. I might add, however, that some food additives may reduce the risk of cancer. The jury is still out on additives, so they should not be condemned outright. Food colorings produce free radicals when they are processed through metabolic chains, thus giving an explanation as to why food colorings should be avoided.

Fifth, excessive consumption of alcoholic beverages, especially with the use of tobacco products, greatly increases the risk of cancer. Smoking alone is also a significant risk factor.

As to specific vitamins and minerals that may confer some level of protection, so far there is sufficient evidence to recommend the beta carotenes, vitamin C, vitamin E, and selenium (up to 200 micrograms per day). Possibly beneficial are copper, iodine, iron, molybdenum, and zinc. However, please note that whereas iron and copper are essential in enzyme systems that scavenge free radicals, both are potent catalysts of free radicals when in the ionic form. As long as the body is slightly deficient in iron and copper there will not be significant amounts of the ionic form. Therefore, supplemental iron or copper should not be used without first confirming that a deficiency exists. A serum ferritin test is needed for the iron, while either erythrocyte copper levels, or a hair analysis (by a reputable laboratory) are preferred for copper. The optimum doses have not been worked out and will be the subject of intense research over the next few decades. The prudent man will not wait that long before changing his habits in line with current knowledge.

It must be re-emphasized, however, that the associations found are with specific classes of food, not food supplements. Whereas there are reasons to believe that the specific nutrients mentioned are the active ones protecting us from cancer, it is most probable that other factors also present in the food, but as yet unrecognized, are the source of the benefits found. This is particularly obvious in the case of fiber: certain types of fiber are more beneficial than others. It may be minerals such as silicon are a factor. Much remains to be discovered.

Cancer seldom attacks without warning, and with early treatment a normal lifespan can be expected. Fear that prevents early diagnosis and treatment is our worst enemy. Worse, in fact, than cancer: those who fear die a thousand deaths, the brave die but once.

Many cancers are caused by abuse: the most glaring examples are lung cancer and all types of skin cancer, the result of smoking and excessive exposure to sunlight, respectively. Yet half of our population prefers to go along with the crowd and ignore the risk until it is too late.

Many cancers occur because we have bypassed the natural methods of preventing those cancers. The most obvious example is the increased colon cancer in those whose diet lacks fiber. But fiber deficiency also promotes cancer of the breast, possibly because toxic substances produced in the colon when wastes are left there too long are absorbed through the colon into the bloodstream. (A high fiber diet helps eliminate toxic peroxidized cholesterol, and also generally is low in fat.) A high fiber diet greatly speeds the transit time from days to mere hours. Fiber is also a major source of silicon; but whether silicon is the answer to why fiber is so effective is as yet unknown.

Some years ago, while I was in the Navy, I had the good fortune to visit the Yale campus. And while we were there, one of the Yale researchers shared with us a piece of his research which to the best of my knowledge has never been made public. He had used phase light photography to photograph living lymphocytes (a type of white blood cell) as they went about their daily routine. As a physician, I was accustomed to seeing lymphocytes as a blue circular cell that apparently just sat there. To ascribe any real activity to the lymphocyte was foreign to my thinking, as it probably is to most physicians. The living lymphocyte, however, is an astounding cell. In a culture containing cancer cells, the lymphocytes could be seen entering *each* cell, going directly to the nucleus of the cell and apparently inspecting it. If the cell were a normal cell, the lyphocyte left just as it entered: through the cell wall. Amazingly, the cell wall which had just opened to allow the lymphocyte into the interior of the cell closed without a trace of the opening. If the cell were cancerous, however, an even more astounding thing happened: the normally spherical lymphocyte pulled back from the nucleus of the cancerous cell, assumed the shape of a torpedo, and plunged deep into the depths of the offending cell's nucleus, immediately exploding and disintegrating both the lymphocyte and the cancerous cell! It is like something out of *Star Wars*. You would have to see it to believe it. The phase photography movie clearly demonstrated this many times.

Very obviously, our bodies have sophisticated mechanisms for destroying cancerous cells, just as we have systems designed to destroy bacteria and viruses. With such a mechanism in daily operation, there must be a need. I believe that we daily produce cancerous cells in the normal routine of repair and reproduction of cells, and the lymphocytes serve to eliminate those cells before they multiply and destroy us.

That being the case, it would appear that cancer is the result not so much of carcinogenic substances producing cancerous cells, as the failure of normal immune mechanisms to eliminate those cells. True, substances which increase the likelihood of mutation of a dividing cell may serve to overwhelm the immune system, but after a few prudent efforts to eliminate the obvious offenders, we should spend our efforts in looking for ways to enhance our natural immune systems, rather than trying to eliminate from our environment every suspect chemical. If we search hard enough, we will find that the world is full of natural carcinogens: they are part of our natural environment. It should be obvious that if a mechanism exists for eliminating cancerous cells soon after they appear, then mild carcenogenic elements within the environment are expected, and should not be feared. Our efforts should be to discover what maintains our natural defenses, and let our bodies handle the problem in its manner. That is not to say that we should not try to avoid the serious offenders, such as tobacco, asbestos, and excessive ultraviolet light. But let's not get in a panic over something that happens to each of us daily. Fear itself may be a potent cause of cancer.

Finally, in 1982, a breakthrough occurred when the National Academy of Sciences announced that certain vitamins and minerals, summarized above, appear to prevent cancer. In fact, these nutrients also seem to help those with cancer to recover: a not-so-surprising finding considering our body's amazing defense systems. Animal studies have proven that the following nutrients prevent cancer in animals, and also will slow the growth of those cancers already present: vitamin A (especially beta carotene), vitamin C, vitamin E, and vitamin B-1 (thiamine), selenium, and zinc. Three of the amino acids (especially cystein) also are beneficial, but should be present in the diet already. The food additives BHT and BHA, both antioxidants, are also greatly beneficial. These last items are a real irony, since one of the results of the efforts of those who have been pushing natural foods has been to eliminate the artificial antioxidants from our foods. The resulting toxins are many more times more dangerous than the purported risks of the antioxidants. We need to balance our enthusiasm with at least some intelligence.

These nutrients act to stimulate the immune system, which normally would be constantly active to rid our bodies of cancer cells. They also are antioxidants, and therefore scavenge free radicals, the primary cause of cancer (and aging and degenerative diseases).

The study discovered that those whose diets include a lot of vegetables and fruit, especially the yellow vegetables, and those with dark green leaves, are much less likely to suffer from cancer. Nutrition, it turns out, will prove in this generation to be our main tool in the prevention of cancer. It may also be our best tool in the cure of cancer, but that remains to be seen.

It must be emphasized that vitamin A, zinc, and selenium are toxic, and can be lethal, if taken to excess. The safe limit of vitamin A is probably as high as 50,000 units daily, although if the beta carotene form is used it will not be toxic since that form is water soluble. The beta carotene is also superior because it is not stored in the liver, but distributes itself throughout the body. In addition, beta carotene is the only scavenger of singlet oxygen, the most active of all free radicals. In fact, singlet oxygen is so potent that your white cells use it to kill bacteria, and have an enzyme to neutralize it. If you have ever used hydrogen peroxide to clean a wound, the foaming action is the effect of your enzymes neutralizing the hydrogen peroxide by transforming it into water and oxygen. Beta carotene is what gives yellow vegetables their color. However, since some diabetics cannot convert the beta carotenes to retinol (the fat soluble vitamin A), both retinol and beta carotene must be consumed. The safe daily limit for zinc is about 60 milligrams daily; however, doses in excess of 45 milligrams daily will block the uptake of copper (which may prove beneficial). This can be partially overcome by taking your zinc at bedtime. For selenium, the limit is about 2000 micrograms daily. A safe and sane dosage would be about 25,000 units of vitamin A (at least 15,000 units as beta carotene), 30 milligrams of zinc, and 300 micrograms of selenium. Before you run out and start dosing yourself with these minerals, it would be best to have a trace mineral hair analysis done to determine your body levels. The soil in some parts of the world have ample of these minerals, and if you take additional supplements, you run the risk of toxic doses.

Incidentally, selenium salts, commonly used in dandruff shampoos, can be absorbed through the skin. Selenium shampoos are sometimes used to treat a certain type of skin fungus, and the manufacturers clearly indicate that the dose should be limited, but I am aware of one man who took whole body shampoos with a selenium shampoo several times daily, and allowed the shampoo to remain on the skin several minutes each time. After about a week, he developed depigmentation of the skin, and a loss of vision from damage to the pigment layer of the retina. His vision recovered. The skin is not an absolute barrier to everything we rub on it. Many things, some toxic, pass through easily.

Dr. Linus Pauling has clearly established that vitamin C, given in dosages of 10 grams daily, prolongs the life of terminal cancer patients by as much as 400 percent. He is now repeating the study with 20 grams daily. My own opinion is that a lower dosage should also be tried, since many people have difficulties with 10 grams of ascorbic acid daily. Perhaps a lower dosage would also be effective.

Currently, I have one patient with a basal cell carinoma which is located where surgery would be especially difficult. After discussing the options, since she refused surgery, we elected to treat it by applying vitamin E plus selenium topically three times daily. The tumor is shrinking. Since the basal cell carcinoma is slow growing and does not metastasize, such a conservative approach is reasonable and safe. I am not recommending this for more malignant tumors, nor for basal cell carcinomas more conveniently located. The point I am making is that a free radical scavenger apparently was able to shrink the size of that particular tumor. If you have a basal cell carcinoma, do not attempt to treat it yourself in this manner. At the very least, work in cooperation with a surgeon who can tell you when its size makes excision mandatory.

Formerly, it was thought that the cancer victim should essentially starve, hoping in the process to also starve the cancer cells. This philosophy has since been proven to be in error, easily recognized when we recall the elaborate defense mechanisms we have to protect ourselves. Starving may deprive cancer cells of vital nutrients. But not many: these cells have the ability to requisition for themselves those nutrients needed, thus leaving the remainder of the body without nutrients needed to defend itself. It is far better to supply the cancer victim with a nutritious diet so that he can defend himself, than it is to starve him in the mistaken notion that the cancer is also being starved. There is no way of depriving the cancer cells of their nutrition short of killing the patient, certainly not the most desirable route to follow. The first line of defense for the cancer victim is good nutrition.

But, surely it is wrong to suggest that diet should be considered when powerful cytotoxic agents are available to destroy cancer cells. No. Because the evidence is clear that in spite of more and more intense therapy with toxic drugs, the overall mortality of the majority of cancer patients has been unchanged over the past twenty-five years. I am not suggesting that cytotoxic agents should be abandoned, but I am suggesting that good nutrition will prove to be far more effective. Cytotoxic agents work against the body's natural defenses, whereas good nutrition works with those defenses. The object with any treatment with cytotoxic drugs is to find that dose which is sufficiently toxic to kill the cancer cells, but is just short of killing the patient. The lethal dose is extremely close to the effective dose. We sometimes lose sight of the fact that the object is to treat the patient, not merely to kill the cancer.

Nutrition is not the whole picture, however. We all are aware of persons who developed cancer soon after a period of severe stress or grief. Knowing the usual mechanisms of defense, and the fact that vitamins A, C, and the mineral zinc are depleted with stress, we can surmise that stress contributes to the development of cancer by reducing the body's defense systems. But there is more to it than this: cancer patients who visualize themselves as fighting a losing or holding action against their cancer will usually die of cancer, while those with positive attitudes and see themselves victorious over the cancer cells usually win the victory. If you see yourself as within a fort holding off the enemy, you probably will eventually lose: even in war holding actions are doomed to failure as it was for the United States in Vietnam. If you see yourself going out and seeking the enemy to destroy them, then your chances of victory are greatly increased. It is not mind over matter: it would appear that each cell in the body can be individually addressed and inspired to great efforts. We are not so much a single body, as a colony of symbiotic organisms. Meditate on that a bit: there is evidence to support the idea. This concept was what I was implying when I suggested that fear of cancer is a possible cause of cancer.

Our choice of foods can overload us with carcinogens, sometimes those foods which would seem to be best are our undoing. Unsaturated oils are a perfect example: recommended to lower cholesterol and reduce the risk of heart attack, they oxidize readily, producing many free radicals. Within the past few months a study was released suggesting that the increase in stomach cancer in the U.S. might be due to oxidized oils used to cook French fries at fast food restaurants. Unsaturated oils oxidize especially fast when heated, and the free radicals appear to be preferentially picked up by the potatoes. (Cooks have long known that frying potatoes will purify rancid oil.) Oxidation of the unsaturated oils could be avoided by the addition of vitamin E to the oils, or by use of synthetic antioxidants such as BHT or BHA. Of course, saturated oils also oxidize, but it takes longer and requires higher temperatures.

It has been argued that unsaturated oils are good sources of vitamin E, and they are. However, except for cottonseed oil, these oils require more vitamin E to protect them from oxidation than they contain, so that the effect is a net loss of vitamin E from the body. Even worse, the high price of vitamin E has made it lucrative to remove the vitamin E from oils before selling the oils, so that the oil you buy is apt to have had its vitamin E removed. So by switching from butter and shortening to margarine and oils, you are increasing your need for vitamin E and decreasing your supply. You may also be increasing your likelihood of getting cancer, and are definitely raising your LDL cholesterol levels. So much for good intensions. Incidentally, since LDL cholesterol levels are an indication of free radical activity, this test should prove a good predictor of the risk of developing a malignancy.

Our family has gotten around the problem by returning to butter instead of margarine, and baking and roasting foods rather than frying. When we fry, we generally use butter, which oxidizes much less readily, and tastes so much better. Butter burns easily, and many do not like to use it for frying. However, by melting butter beforehand, and skimming off the foam floating at the top, you obtain a clear "butter" which will not burn (nor oxidize), but still has the good flavor you desire. An alternate is to use spray products such as PAM™.

If you fry bacon or hamburgers, throw away the grease. Use a lower temperature and do not overcook. Grilling meat also produces a lot of free radicals, especially from the grease burning on the hot coals. An enclosed grill, where the meat is not directly over the fire, will greatly reduce the risk. There is a newer design gas grill that uses intense infrared heat from above the meat, so that the dripping grease does not burn. This type works very well for steaks, but not for ground meats which are difficult to turn without breaking the pattie apart.

Oxidation is reduced by cooking at lower temperatures. Thus boiling, stewing, slow cooking in a slow cooker, or cooking in a microwave oven are much preferred over frying or grilling. If you grill, and we do, use a lower heat setting so that the grease drippings do not flame up, and so that the meat cooks more slowly and does not burn. Using an enclosed grill and placing the meat away from the heat will also help. The infrared type gas grill avoids many of these problems.

Evening primrose oil, taken six capsules per day, has been very effective in producing remission in terminal cancer patients in studies in England and Australia. Since L-Carnitine boosts the effect of Evening primrose oil, and margarine blocks these beneficial effects, margarine should be discontinued, and L-Carnitine taken.

Incidentally, Evening primrose oil and L-Carnitine tend to produce a gradual weight loss.

Thirty-five percent food grade hydrogen peroxide, taken in gradually increasing doses of from 1 to 4 drops per glass of drink (water or juice) is claimed by some to cure some cancers and free radical diseases. Taken as directed, it is safe. Absolutely do not use regular hydrogen peroxide, and use only diluted food grade products.

Coenzyme Q10 and N,N Dimethylglycine have been proven effective in animal studies in preventing cancer. Certainly their use in human cancer should be considered since they are non-toxic. I am also aware of a few patients with terminal cancer who went into remission upon use of Body Toddy™, 4 ounces per day. Body Toddy™ is an excellent source of selenium, proven to be effective against cancer.

In summary, cancer is best prevented by avoiding those known potent carcinogens, plus eating a nutritious diet rich in vegetables, and supplemented with those elements (all of which are free radical scavengers) proven to reduce the incidence of cancer. Cast out all fear. Fear not only will weaken your defenses against cancer and all illnesses, but fear will make you more susceptible to that which you fear. Those who have lived in constant fear of cancer, have frequently died of cancer. If cancer is suspected, early diagnosis and treatment are your best defense, followed by good nutrition and a positive attitude. If possible, have your treatment monitored by a physician who knows all treatment modalities available, and will help you balance cost and risk against the possibility of a cure and a useful life. There is no real advantage in gaining three more months of life if those months are spent ill from effects of treatment. Death is not the end: it is the beginning, a graduation to greater things. No treatment has ever prevented death, but only delayed the inevitable. What you do in the interim is what makes the effort worthwhile. When Jesus told his disciples to take up their cross and follow him, he was not telling them that they had a burden to bear. Jesus clearly said that he would bear our burden; we do not have to bear it. In that day, a man carrying his cross would be dead by nightfall. Jesus was telling his disciples that they should live each day as though that was their last day on Earth. If you live that way, you will find each day is a blessing, and you will dispense with a lot of frivolous things.

XV.
A Sane Approach to Free Radicals

Free radical pathology is discussed under several topics in this book, for the simple reason that free radical pathology is very possibly the key to so many degenerative diseases. In general, a free radical is a molecule or atom which has an unpaired electron in its outer electron shell, making it extremely reactive. A free radical might be thought of as an accident looking for a place to happen. Of the free radicals, singlet oxygen is the most reactive. A free radical compound will react with any available molecule. If that molecule plays a key role as an enzyme, structural molecule, or genetic material, then the damage can be severe. Obviously, the majority of free radical reactions are inconsequential, or we would die instantly, as we indeed will if the free radical density becomes too great. In fact, that is exactly the cause of death in a heart attack or radiation sickness. Since free radicals catalyse free radicals, (that is, they tend to create more free radicals) the problem of controlling their density is critical. Rather than stand in fear, you need to formulate your own program to avoid, and reverse, free radical pathology. Fortunately, within limits, our bodies are able to repair free radical damage, given time, relief from free radical bombardment, and suitable building blocks for repair. It is not the intention of this chapter to repeat everything scattered throughout the other chapters in this book, but to summarize sensible and practical approaches to combat free radical pathology, approaches that are apt to be followed.

First, how can you tell if you have free radical damage? The truth is, everyone has such damage, even those who carefully plan to minimize that damage. I seriously doubt that free radical pathology can be totally eliminated. However, there are a few simple ways in which you can determine whether the damage you have already sustained is severe. One simple test is to look at your ear lobe in the mirror: if you have a crease across the lobe, you already have very significant cross linkage of collagen, one sign of free radical pathology. Wrinkles in the skin are also signs of cross linkage. Those brown age spots on the skin are also evidence of free radical pathology. Hold your hand in front of you, palm down, then grasp the skin on the back of your hand in a fold and lift gently, then release crisply. Healthy elastic skin (without free radical pathology) will snap back instantly. Do this to someone under 20 years of age to see how normal skin should react. If your skin slowly slides back into place, count yourself a victim of free radical pathology. If it is still folded several seconds later, then your damage is fairly advanced. If you have any of the degenerative diseases of aging, including hypertension, arthritis, diabetes, aging, senility, Alzheimer's, atherosclerosis, stroke, glaucoma, cataracts, cancer, loss of memory, and sensory loss (hearing, taste, smell), you most probably have already suffered considerable damage. Finally, an easy assessment of free radical activity can be had by measuring blood cholesterol, plus the LDL and HDL fractions. An elevated LDL cholesterol is proof of free radical activity. A low blood cholesterol with a high HDL fraction is an indication that you are doing something right. All of these signs and symptoms are reversible to a greater or lesser degree.

Let us review the sources of free radicals: 1) anoxia, 2) unsaturated fats, 3) fats in general, 4) radiation, 5) ionized iron and copper, 6) toxic metals, including cadmium and aluminum, 7) complex hydrocarbons (smog and pollution), 8) tobacco smoke, 9) food additives, 10) alcohol, and 11) free radicals. Any one of these factors, either alone or in concert, can catalyse or generate free radicals.

Anoxia produces free radicals. While you are sitting around watching TV, reading this book, or writing as I am now, portions of your body are becoming relatively anoxic. Since free radicals encourage the coagulation of blood, any anoxia will tend to produce a thrombosis. And since the rupture of blood cells in a blood clot releases iron and copper, more free radicals are generated which tend to extend the thrombosis. It does not take a genius to figure that cardiac anoxia can set up a sequence of events that can kill you. In the legs, the resulting thrombophlebitis can release an embolus which can go to the lungs and be fatal. This correlation is also the reason why large doses of vitamin E and the other antioxidant compounds mentioned below are preferred therapy for thrombotic disease. Thrombosis is the result of a free radical crisis.

The best way to combat anoxia is physical activity: good, prolonged, regular physical exercise. Obviously, smoking not only produces anoxia, but provides its own free radical catalysts, and in addition speeds clotting time for blood. This is definitely not a good combination of conditions. Periodically getting up and walking around will reduce the risk of anoxia-induced free radical pathology.

Harvard University released a study showing that even moderate exercise, such as walking, engaged in for thirty minutes at a time for several days a week on a regular basis, is effective in prolonging life. It doesn't take jogging five miles every day to get benefits from exercise.

All fats, when they oxidize, produce lipid peroxides which are free radicals. Unsaturated fats oxidize almost immediately upon being pressed out of their source and being exposed to the air. Cold pressing, highly touted by health food stores, has no lasting advantage over standard manufacturing methods. The only way oil could be extracted without oxidation would be to do it under an inert atmosphere of nitrogen, and to then add sufficient amounts of antioxidants to the oil to prevent its subsequent oxidation. Needless to say, banning removal of vitamin E from food grade oils would be a great step forward. Of the available oils, only cottonseed oil and olive oil have any possibility of having low levels of lipid peroxides. The situation is made worse by the fact that manufacturers are removing vitamin E from oils (which would protect them from oxidation) for sale separately. Saturated fats peroxidize less rapidly, and are therefore less likely to produce free radicals. Butter is therefore much to be preferred over any margarine, or any vegetable oil.

Fatty tissue within the body also randomly forms lipid peroxides, which hopefully are neutralized before damage occurs. Nevertheless, the more fat you have in your body, the greater the number of free radicals produced internally. Free radical pathology goes far to explain why obesity is associated with so many degenerative diseases.

Getting rid of all your excess fat is an obvious way to reduce your free radical burden. I refer you to the chapter on weight control for a fuller discussion.

Since fats form lipid peroxides most easily when exposed to heat and oxygen, avoid fried foods whenever possible. The worst type of fried food will be fried in oils which have been repeatedly used for frying, such as you might do to save money, or as is routinely done at fast food restaurants. If you must fry, use a saturated fat such as butter, beef suet, or vegetable shortening, since these oxidize less readily than unsaturated vegetable oils.

(Unfortunately, vegetable shortening is a modified fat, and produces cellular membrane damage by another mechanism.) Similarly, fats dripping on hot charcoal are instantly oxidized, giving us the charcoal flavor we love. Unfortunately, the taste we love is lipid peroxides.

Since unsaturated fats (typically vegetable oils) oxidize so rapidly, purchase them in small quantities in glass bottles, and add an antioxidant such as BHT to prevent further oxidation. Durk Pearson and Sandy Shaw, authors of the book *Life Extension*, recommend one teaspoon per quart of oil, which is ten times the amount permitted by the FDA. You will have to come to your own mind on this, and decide whether the peroxidized oil is more dangerous than the BHT. The answer to that question is unknown at the present time. One way to find out whether adding BHT is beneficial is to have your LDL cholesterol measured before and after using the antioxidant for several months. If your LDL levels drop, then you are effective in controlling your free radicals. Obviously, studies need to be made in this area.

Increased surface area, plus heat, increases the potential for lipid peroxidation. An ideal combination to develop this unfortunate combination is ground meat, which mixes fat with ionized iron and copper (from the blood) and air, producing rapid oxidation. Buy your hamburger fresh, and use it promptly. Pay the extra to buy lean ground meat. In an ideal world, you would grind your own hamburger and cook it immediately.

Radiation induced free radicals are discussed elsewhere. Their neutralization is the same as for any other free radical. Needless to say, avoid X-rays unless necessary. Your doctor may have to take an X-ray to protect himself from a malpractice suit, even though he is certain of the diagnosis without this test. Although the amount of radiation from modern equipment is reduced from that previously produced, all unnecessary radiation should be avoided. Consuming foods with beta cartotene and taking perhaps 1000 units of vitamin E and 1000 milligrams of vitamin C about thirty minutes before radiation exposure will significantly reduce damage from radiation.

Since ionized iron and copper are potent free radical catalysts, their excess should be avoided. Keeping yourself slightly iron deficient would be a reasonable approach. This can be accomplished by avoiding iron supplements unless you have a documented deficiency, and by donating blood regularly to the blood bank. Three units donated per year would effectively keep you slightly iron deficient, and thus free from ionized iron. Women have no need to take this extra precaution prior to menopause. Likewise, copper supplements should not be taken unless you have confirmed a need by laboratory tests (erythrocyte copper levels or a hair analysis). If you are building, avoid copper plumbing if your water is soft or acidic. Zinc supplements can be used to reduce your copper uptake. If you really have a problem with iron or copper, chelation therapy is strongly advised to quickly remove the excess iron and copper ions.

Chelation is by far the most efficient method for removing toxic metals of whatever type. Vitamin C and zinc supplements are also helpful in helping speed the excretion of some of these metals. In fact, supplementation with any metal trace element will inhibit the uptake of other metal ions, so supplementation is strongly advised. Most toxic metals can be detected by hair analysis.

Aluminum toxicity will be difficult to avoid, since aluminum is added to so many processed foods. Beverages stored in aluminum containers probably will pick up aluminium ions, but whether toxic amounts are dissolved is not yet known. Certainly, cooking foods that require prolonged cooking times in aluminum vessels is to be avoided: use stainless steel instead unless the aluminum container is Teflon™ coated. However, the amount of aluminum from aluminum cooking vessels is meager when compared to the amount of aluminum being ingested as food additives and antacid tablets, or absorbed through the skin from cosmetics and antiperspirant drugs. If data concerning aluminum's role in Alzheimer's disease, loss of memory, and Parkinson's disease is correct, we are setting ourselves up for a sociological disaster a few short years from now. I believe the evidence is strong enough that the prudent person will eliminate *all* food and cosmetic sources of aluminum, and will use aluminum cooking utensils only if they are coated. Since aluminum salts bind phosphorus, we may be fortunate that our dietary excess phosphorus has bound much of the aluminum we have ingested. We may have accidently protected ourselves from both excesses. Chelation therapy is the most efficient method of removing aluminum from the body. It may be the only way.

Complex hydrocarbons, including both smog and tobacco smoke, produce free radicals during the detoxification process. Since vitamin E is the first line of defense against free radical pathology, it is understandable why this vitamin has proved effective in combating lung damage due to atmospheric pollutants. Obviously, the best way to deal with pollution is to avoid it, and not generate your own. Practicing conservation of energy will reduce pollution, but may not benefit you directly. Installing an electrostatic filter in your house will remove particulate pollutants, but having a tightly sealed house will cause a significant increase in pollution within your home. This age of superinsulation is producing indoor pollution far exceeding allowable outdoor limits. Take advantage of mild weather to air out your home, and if you are building, consider a system that exchanges indoor air with outdoor air while conserving heat. Use exhaust fans to eliminate high concentrations of pollution, such as occur in the kitchen while cooking. Unfortunately, other than avoiding tobacco smoke (first or second hand) or moving to a South Sea island, we are stuck with pollution. When you vote, you might consider environmental issues at least as strongly as you do their dollar cost.

Food additives should be avoided whenever possible, except those additives that inhibit oxidation, such as BHA, BHT, vitamin C, and vitamin E. Food colorings, apparently added to almost everything, are especially to be avoided. This advice is more easily said than done, but can be approached by preparing your food from scratch whenever possible, and avoiding highly processed foods. If you have a choice between a food which has added iron (or vitamins), choose the one without the added supplements. Having a home garden is an excellent way if you tend to practice organic techniques, and minimize use of insecticides. We are now into the fourth year of gardening without pesticides, and insect damage is virtually nil. Pesticides also kill predatory insects which work overtime to keep your garden pests under control. We also take advantage companion planting, and plants which discourage pests.

Finally, alcohol is metabolized to acetaldehyde, which oxidizes within the body in the presence of unsaturated lipids (fats) to produce a virtual explosion of free radicals. Our bodies contain enzymes to detoxify acetaldehyde, but more than a couple of drinks can overwhelm this protective system. Alcohol in moderation, however, tends to produce favorable HDL cholesterol levels. Like iron, a little is good for you, too much is deadly. Notice that the combination of excess alcohol with a diet rich in unsaturated fats is fairly a guarantee of free radical pathology.

Having done all of the above, you will have only reduced your free radical burden. You will not have neutralized it. This requires some knowledge about how the body is organized to control free radical pathology, a rather elaborate and amazing system. Since a free radical is a highly reactive molecule looking for an opportunity to react, and since a free radical produces damage only if it reacts with a critical body component (whether enzyme, genetic material, or cell membrane), then damage control consists in providing those free radicals with opportunities to react harmlessly. However, even this approach has its limitations, since the number of free radicals is almost unlimited. The solution is to provide a means of regenerating the reacting (neutralizing) compound after it has reacted with a free radical.

This logical approach is exactly what our bodies use. Beta carotene, found most plentifully in dark and yellow vegetables, will effectively neutralize the most destructive free radical, singlet oxygen. In fact, beta carotene seems to be our only defense against this particular free radical.

Vitamin E is the first line of defense against all other free radicals whether from pollution, or generated internally (but outside the mitochondria). In the process, vitamin E is converted to tocoperol quinone. Oxidized vitamin E is recycled to tocoperol (reduced vitamin E) by vitamin C, which in turn is oxidized in the reaction to dehydroascorbate. A selenium-containing enzyme, glutathione peroxidase, restores vitamin C to its former activity. Cysteine, an essential amino acid, is used in the synthesis of glutathione peroxidase. Gluthathione peroxidase must then oxidize glutathione to be recycled, and the oxidized glutathione, in turn, is reduced (the opposite of oxidation) back to glutathione by the enzyme glutathione reductase. This last reaction requires the vitamin riboflavin. Another B vitamin, niacin, is involved in the reaction which restores the activity of glutathione reductase. At this point, the chain of reactions enters a metabolic pathway which results in energy production for useful work. It is rather astounding, isn't it, that our body extracts energy from pollution? It may also partially explain why some of us gain weight after beginning on a supplement program.

Selenium, in addition to acting as part of the enzyme glutathione peroxidase, is a potent free radical scavenger by itself. Selenium is toxic in excess, but you can safely consume 200-2000 micrograms daily and use it profitably. Since the soil in some parts of the country is rich in selenium, a hair analysis at a reputable laboratory is indicated before beginning use of selenium, and after several months of taking high does of selenium.

Chromium and vanadium both are effective in reducing blood cholesterol levels, which indicates that they have some free radical inhibiting property. This effect might be indirect. For example, chromium is effective in lowering blood sugar, and sugar competes with vitamin C for a blood protein transport mechanism.

A lowered blood sugar would result in more vitamin C distributed throughout the body, and thus more effective neutralization of free radicals.

As mentioned in an earlier chapter, free radicals are used in the production of energy in the carefully controlled environment of the mitochondria. These free radicals are then neutralized by the enzyme, superoxide dismutase (SOD), which contains manganese as its active metal ion. Manganese is typically deficient in the American diet, and should be supplemented. Twenty milligrams daily of chelated manganese would be sufficient. If dietary manganese is deficient, free radicals from within the mitochondria will escape, providing the major source of single oxygen within the body, which must then be dealt with outside the mitochondria. Another form of superoxide dismutase (SOD) is normally present outside the mitochondria, and this form of the SOD requires both zinc and copper in its makeup. Zinc can be taken as much as 45 milligrams per day, but I would advise that if you are taking more than 20 milligrams, take the extra as a separate nighttime dose just before retiring to prevent interference with absorption of other elements. Zinc is toxic if more than 60 milligrams per day is taken. Zinc also blocks copper uptake if more than 45 milligrams are taken along with copper. This can be used to your advantage if you have a copper excess, which will in itself generate free radicals.

Since singlet oxygen is the most devastating free radical, and since the most effective scavenger of singlet oxygen is beta carotene, and since beta carotene is water soluble, you will need to include foods rich in beta carotene in your daily diet. The yellow vegetables and fruit, plus the dark green leafy vegetables (and especially broccoli) are your best sources of necessary beta carotene. Since this valuable pro-vitamin is destroyed by heat, these vegetables should be cooked very little, and with minimal water. Steaming or using a microwave oven is ideal.

Both onions and garlic contain antioxidant compounds, as do all the members of the cabbage family. An ideal food, from this point of view, is sliced squash and chopped onions cooked together with a small amount of salt and pepper or spices, and butter if desired. Cooked onion and garlic both retain their anti free radical effect, and are certainly less offensive. Include either onions or garlic in every meal, and especially if the meal is a fatty one.

Another potent antioxidant food is a carrot and cabbage slaw. There are ample ideas of ways to include these wholesome vegetables in your daily diet.

Refined flour and sugar are depleted of micronutrients normally present in the natural food. Consumption of these refined foods greatly stresses the body's ability to use its food and defend itself against free radicals. I would strongly recommend eliminating sugar from your diet, along with white flour and white flour products. While it is true that you can take supplements and protect yourself from most of the damage these products impose, it is also highly probable that unrefined flour contains nutrients as yet unidentified.

Insofar as possible, eat whole foods (they have more nutrients, and are less likely to be oxidized). In addition, whole foods generally contain more fiber, and fiber is necessary for the body to eliminate toxic peroxidized cholesterol. As a side benefit, whole foods require more chewing, and chewing is an effective adjunct to a weight control program.

Cholesterol, in its reduced form, is not toxic, and is very beneficial. In fact, it reacts freely with free radicals and neutralizes their effect. Reduced cholesterol, the type measured by the HDL fraction, has as one of its major functions the control of free radical damage. Egg yolks are rich in cholesterol, but remember if the egg yolk is broken during the cooking process, the cholesterol is rapidly oxidized to its toxic form. Therefore prepare your eggs boiled, poached, or sunnyside up with the yolk intact. Avoid eggs scrambled, in omelets, or added to recipes as part of a mixture.

Is a supplement approach such as outlined above effective? Very definitely! Even while eating my eggs scrambled, and depriving myself of sufficient exercise, my use of such a supplement program dropped my cholesterol levels by over 30 percent within six months. It is so effective, in fact, that an occasional indiscretion will not derail your program. In any case, you will be far better off than you were before you began.

If you have begun later in life (perhaps past age 35) with a program of preventive maintenance, seriously consider chelation therapy as an effective means of reversing free radical pathology, which it does by removing toxic heavy metal ions, plus other metal ions (iron and copper) which catalyse free radicals. I strongly urge you to study the chapter on chelation, and also obtain and study the book, *Bypassing Bypass*, by Dr. Elmer Cranton. The information contained therein, if acted upon, can greatly prolong your useful life.

Finally, include a generous supply of fresh fruit in your diet. By growing many of our own fruit, we have discovered a beautiful plan in the pattern of ripening fruit. Strawberries ripen early, and continue until you are tired of them, at which time the blueberries are in season. The blueberry season overlaps with the peaches, which overlaps with the pear season. Finally, apples bring the bountiful harvest season to a close. When we lived in Japan we became accustomed to seasonal fruit and vegetables, and ate them greedily while they were in season. By the time we were tired of one fruit, it was no longer available, and a new fruit came into season. Fruit in season is always much fresher and flavorful than fruit stored for a year, regardless of how well it is stored. In addition, your appetite for a certain fruit will have been whetted by the long wait for the fruit to again be available. We in America have certainly lost a lot as a result of giant corporations controlling our food production and distribution. Not only have we lost a lot of our nutrition, but the annual joy of a friend revisited as a favorite fruit returns to the market. We have also lost a lot of flavor as unripe fruit is picked early so that it will store for a long time, then artificially colored to appear ripe. Tomatoes are a classical example: those who have eaten home grown tomatoes are not fooled by the inferior commercial product available in most stores.

At some point you must decide whether such a program is worth the cost. The cost in vitamin and mineral supplements will be less than 75 cents per day, even for an aggressive program. If you smoke or drink carbonated beverages regularly, you are already spending more than that to harm your health. By switching to preparing food from scratch, and avoiding fast food restaurants, you will save far more than the cost of supplements. Since it is estimated that the cost of medical care could be cut to less than half by proper nutrition, you can figure on a savings of about $1000 per family per year in health care costs. It may be more than that, since it has been calculated that the additional cost incurred by the smoker averages $3.50 per pack of cigarettes, but now paid by all of us. My success rate in reversing cataracts and avoiding surgery is better than 50 percent. Since each person who avoids cataract surgery saves about $8000, figure how many days you can take the recommended supplement program for that savings. Even considering the 50 percent efficiency, that comes to eighteen and one-half years worth of supplements. And we are still ignoring savings in other medical bills such as for time spent in a coronary intensive care unit, or in a skilled nursing home facility as a result of senility. The truth is, nutritional therapy does not cost, it pays. And it pays more dividends if the investment is made earlier in life. The return in additional productive years gained is priceless.

Finally, you must be aware that drugs you take in treatment of free radical-induced disease will not be needed as much after your free radical density is controlled. This is especially true of anticoagulant drugs (blood thinners) used to prevent the thrombosis caused by free radicals. The program proposed here can convert a maintenance dose to a lethal dose. Discontinuing anticoagulants suddenly is not the answer, because that may precipitate a thrombosis. You must work with your physician in adjusting your dosage as your supplemental program becomes effective. Likewise, antihypertensive drugs may require a lower dose to avoid complications. I especially warn my diabetic patients on insulin to monitor their sugar levels carefully for several months after beginning such a program.

Another powerful antioxidant recently commercially available is Coenzyme Q10. This enzyme is part of our energy production system, and can be produced internally in presence of adequate vitamin E and selenium (both typically deficient). In animal studies Coenzyme Q10 prolongs lifespan by as much as 56 percent. Fortunately, it is stored within the body and recycled, so that large doses do not have to be taken daily. It would appear that a reasonable approach to its use would be to take 30 to 300 milligrams daily for about 3000 milligrams, and if you note any major improvement in your general health, continue at 30 milligrams per day indefinitely. If my clinical experience is any indication, then there will be no question about whether or not you are having good results. Coenzyme Q10 is totally non-toxic.

XVI.
Chelation Therapy·

Most of the vitamins and minerals associated with improved resistance to cancer and reduced aging also turn out to be chelates. A chelate is a substance which attaches itself to another molecule making it soluble. The word itself is Greek for "claw," and graphically portrays what the chelate actually does, grasping and seizing the ion or molecule to the chelated.

All life depends upon chelates. Digestion and assimilation of nutrients depend upon chelation so that ordinarily insoluble substances can pass through the walls of the intestines into the bloodsteam. Minerals which have been added to the nutrient broth for yeast become chelated, and therefore more easily assimilated than non-chelated minerals when used in a supplement. Assuming there is no allergy to yeast products, there are fewer side effects. Some minerals necessary for life are of no benefit unless they are in a chelated form. In fact, some enzymes and vitamins are trace element chelates.

Chelation is the method of action of many of the drugs used today, from antibiotics to pain medications. Chelates are rather specific as to which ion they attract and bind, so there are literally thousands of chelates used daily in medicine and industry. Chelation is absolutely necessary for life and health, both naturally and therapeutically.

The fact that nutritional therapy is effective in restoring health is largely due to chelation by the relatively weak natural chelates. Were our diet to have sufficient amounts of these substances, chelation therapy with stronger synthetic substances would not be necessary. Nevertheless, chelation therapy by dietary supplementation is effective, albeit slow.

EDTA is a synthetic amino acid first used in human therapy in 1947. It has a strong affinity for metal ions, and will "drop" one ion if another is available for which it has a higher affinity. The order of affinity, from highest to lowest, is: chromium 2+, iron 3+, mercury 2+, copper 2+, lead 2+, zinc 2+, cadmium 2+, cobalt 2+, aluminum 3+, iron 2+, manganese 2+, calcium 2+, and magnesium 2+. By delivering EDTA as magnesium EDTA, the chelating physician is not only removing toxic metal ions, but administering magnesium which is apt to be deficient. Other deficiencies can be corrected in the same way, but obviously if chromium EDTA were administered, only chromium EDTA would be excreted. Except for chromium and zinc, most of the ions for which EDTA has a high affinity are toxic heavy metals, or those which catalyse free radical reactions. Given intravenously, it will remove those ions by chelation and excretion through the kidneys. It will also remove some beneficial ions, such as zinc and chromium, and these will have to be replaced. It has been used intravenously safely over six million times in over 400,000 patients in the United States alone. Its success rate in restoring circulation to clogged arteries appoaches 82 percent, with less risk, greater effectiveness, and at one-tenth the cost of vascular surgery.

It is uncertain just how chelation works, but there is speculation that EDTA binds excess iron and copper (plus toxic heavy metals), thus preventing much free radical activity. It appears that it is this inhibition of free radical activity that allows the body's natural healing processes to repair the damage from free radical pathology. Another interesting discovery is that lactic acid is a chelating agent. Lactic acid is produced during vigorous exercise, and its action as a chelating agent may explain why exercise is so beneficial. Unfortunately, most patients requiring chelation therapy have allowed their physical condition to deteriorate so far that exercise is almost impossible. If you establish a regular exercise program and stick with it, it is likely you can avoid both bypass surgery and chelation. But you will not avoid the need to reduce free radical damage by use of nutritional therapy.

Is EDTA safe? Go to your pantry, and you will see that you consume EDTA with almost any food you eat. It is added to virtually all processed foods to stabilize them and prevent spoilage. It is also used in shampoos, detergents, water softeners, and an amazingly long list of products. EDTA is safe. EDTA does not pass readily through the walls of the intestines, so that oral consumption is not effective for internal chelation. It is effective, though, in preventing metal ions in food from being absorbed. Used intravenously, it has a therapeutic index far superior to aspirin. (The therapeutic index is a measure of safety.)

EDTA chelation therapy is usually performed by physicians who themselves resorted to it when their options in life finally ran out. Their successful recovery has made them a rather enthusiastic group. Unfortunately, these courageous physicians perform this service to others at great personal risk, since organized medicine has generally been against this mode of therapy. This has put the chelation therapists at great risk of legal action and the loss of their license to practice medicine, although as physicians they certainly have the right to do what is best for their patients. Health insurance generally will not pay for treatments, which cost about $100 for each of the at least twenty or more treatments needed. Such costs are a force against the use of this type of therapy.

There are risks if it is infused too fast, but decades of experience have virtually eliminated this risk if the administering physician has followed the proper protocol. (Full information is available from the American Academy of Medical Preventics (AAMP), 6151 West Century Blvd., Suite 1114, Los Angeles, CA 90045. Their telephone is (213) 645-5350.) Physicians interested in this mode of therapy are strongly advised to follow the training and treatment protocols, and to earn their certificate of qualification. Patients who are interested in chelation therapy, are even more strongly advised to seek only the services of chelation physicians certified by this academy. Just as with every profession, medicine has its few bad eggs, and some have gone into production line chelation. Properly done, chelation takes at least three and one-half hours per treatment, and there is no way to shorten that time safely. Some few clinics (chelation mills might be a better name) are pushing infusion rates to the limits of toleration in order to increase profits. It is important that both concerned physicians and patients take an open stand against such practices now before these few charlatans destroy chelation before it gets a chance to become an accepted mode of therapy.

Actually, chelation with EDTA has been used by physicians for thirty years. Unlike the current rash of drugs, EDTA is cheap and its patent has long since run out. Its safety record is beyond dispute by anyone who cares to look at the record. The only question should be whether it is effective. Again, there is ample evidence that chelation therapy is effective. The fact is that those physicians who are using chelation themselves resorted to chelation when all other options leading to life fell through. Their recovery resulted in their becoming active, even zealous, in chelation therapy.

I do not wish to lay on organized medicine the burden that it is mercenary, nor that it does not care for the best interests of its patients. Nor do I believe that there is an organized attempt to suppress new treatments such as those proposed in this book. In this respect some of my friends say that I am naive, but my experience is that most physicians are much too busy to get involved at that petty level of politics. Physicians are human, though, and some rascals do seem to have made it through the rigors of medical training. Therefore, I am not surprised that an occasional individual will play upon his colleagues' ignorance in enlisting their support to his benefit. Truth, however, will always win in the end and our goal should always be to be on the winning side of truth. *Nevertheless, nutritional and chelation therapy threatens to substantially reduce the cost of health care, translate that "profits," and those who oppose this approach need to give cause why they should be believed. They have a major financial interest in your continuing in poor health, and especially in your submitting to their mode of therapy.*

Pharmaceutical firms, especially, have such a financial interest, and simply will not spend money investigating a substance that has no potential for their profit. Nor should we expect them to. Congress has recognized this partially through the orphan drug bill. EDTA and DMSO fall into this category since they are orphan drugs, and cannot be protected for the benefit of any one company. Since a sizable portion of research dollars comes from these companies, it is not surprising that little research has been done at the major medical centers who survive on those grants. In fact, not only is there no profit in these options, this approach to health would result in a substantial loss of profits to the major pharmaceutical firms. No, do not expect a lot of support from organized medicine, nor from their benefactors.

I do not currently perform chelation therapy, but am convinced that it might prove useful in certain eye diseases, especially macular degeneration and other vascular eye diseases. It is probable that in the best interests of my patients' health, I will someday obtain the additional training necessary to perform this service. Currently, I am studying the options, so to speak, and have not fully committed myself. I am sufficiently convinced that it is only a matter of time before I submit myself to the services of a chelation physician. And that time will be fairly soon.

For those who wish to read a well-documented book on chelation therapy, I would like to recommend *Bypassing Bypass* listed in the list of recommended reading at the end of this book. It is your right to be well-informed, and to demand only the best for yourself. This book is written by Dr. Elmer Cranton, a physician with both academic and practical credentials sufficient to merit a fair hearing. Of the various books written on chelation therapy, this is the most current, and certainly the most informative. It is written to both the general public and practicing physician. It is not a book on how to administer chelation therapy. Any physician who dismisses the advantages of chelation therapy without giving the evidence a fair hearing does not have your best interests at heart.

Note: Since the first printing of this book, I have undergone eighteen chelation treatments. All of the effects I have noted have been beneficial. Among the fellow patients who underwent chelation therapy with me were many with severe circulatory problems whose health visibly improved during their course of treatment. Note that these were patients whose options in life had all run out. As had mine.

XVII.
The Vitamins

Vitamin C

DAILY ALLOWANCES:
  Infants   35 mg.
  Children   40 mg.
  Adults   60 mg.
MAJOR SOURCES:
  Citrus fruit
  Rose hips
  Green peppers
  Broccoli
  Spinach
  Tomatoes
MAJOR BENEFITS:
  Antioxidant (recycles vitamin E)
  Hormone production
  Collagen formation (tendons, scars, ligaments)
  Tooth, bone, and cartilage formation
  Improves iron absorption
  Enhances the ability to fight infection
  Reduces capillary permeability
  Improves capillary strength
  Anticancer effect (part of antioxidant effect)
  Helps reduce levels of toxic oxidized cholesterol
  Helps remove toxic heavy metals from the body
  Necessary for wound healing
  Anti-stress factor

Vitamin C played an important role in the defeat of Napoleon at Waterloo. Before it was discovered that citrus fruit would protect from scurvy, the navies of the world were never able to operate at full force, because vitamin C deficiency would incapacitate the men within two or three months at sea. Only about one third of the average crew were able to man the fleet at any given time. The British discovered that limes would prevent scurvy, and this discovery had the effect of almost instantly making their navy supreme. British sailors are called limies to this day. Being able to break the three-month barrier was as important in that day as breaking free into space has been to our generation.

Scurvy can occur whenever the diet is deficient in vitamin C for more than about sixty days, depending on how much vitamin C the body has stored. The first cases of scurvy I saw were two children during my internship. Later, when I had the privilege of being assigned as medical officer aboard a nuclear submarine, little did I expect to find scurvy in the nuclear navy, but it was there. The only crewmen who developed scurvy were those bachelors whose lifestyles consisted of suds, sand, and the beach life. Not much vitamin C there. Even these did not develop scurvy until several weeks had passed without fresh vegetables. Their classic vitamin C deficiency responded quickly to vitamin replacement.

Blood levels of vitamin C peak with an intake of about 125 milligrams daily. However, storage of vitamin C increases at least until 500 milligrams of vitamin C are ingested daily. The optimum dose of vitamin C is unknown, although studies with guinea pigs suggest that exposure to stress increases the requirement to at least 1500 milligrams per day. Some severe stress situations, such as appendicitis or abdominal surgery, demand as much as 10 grams of vitamin C daily to maintain normal blood levels. Since normal vitamin C stores is about 2 grams, we may conclude that most surgical patients are borderline scorbutic within a day after surgery. And since it has been amply proven that vitamin C deficiency is the usual cause of wound rupture, there is absolutely no excuse not to supplement *every* surgical patient with several grams of vitamin C daily both before and after surgery. I am not alone in this contention, a recent article on healing in a surgical journal takes the same position.

I began using about 250 milligrams of vitamin C daily with my surgical eye patients about twelve years ago, and have never had a spontaneous wound rupture after surgery. I have had one traumatic rupture. Another ophthalmologist I know has as many as five a year. Wound leakage after eye surgery is a milder form of wound rupture, and is all too common. I have yet to have even a wound leak in any patient who was taking vitamin C.

Vitamin C is water soluble, and is quickly excreted via the kidneys. Peak levels are reached within an hour, and return to pre-ingestion levels within about four hours. According to Dr.

Linus Pauling, the beneficial effects of vitamin C are more related to minimum blood levels than to the peak levels, so that optimum dosage would require taking vitamin C at about four-hour intervals. Sustained release tablets alleviate this problem, but cause gas in some persons. Also, dissolution of sustained release tablets is variable. However, if sustained release tablets do not cause you discomfort, they are a good way to maintain high average blood levels of the vitamin.

Vitamin C is an antioxidant, and therefore effective in scavenging free radicals. It also recycles vitamin E, which is the body's primary defense against free radical damage. It is probably this role of vitamin C that makes maintaining high blood levels so important. Dr. Linus Pauling has shown in a careful study that life expectancy of terminal cancer patients is greatly increased with ingestion of 10 grams of vitamin C daily. Dr. Pauling is currently doing a study using 20 grams of vitamin C daily.

I have one glaucoma patient whose glaucoma had been unresponsive to all medications available, but whose pressures were normal on 10 grams of vitamin C daily in divided doses. After a year, she became intolerant of the dose, and it had to be discontinued. This method of treating glaucoma was pioneered by Italian physicians about a decade ago.

Massive doses of vitamin C are being used to cure heroin addiction without withdrawal symptoms. The treatment requires about 10 grams a day for several days. I know of one patient with shingles (a very painful viral disease) whose pain could not be relieved by less than heroic means. A physician mutual friend infused 25 grams of vitamin C intravenously, which stopped the pain almost instantly, and maintained him pain-free for several hours. This was repeated several times before the pain did not return. It would be interesting to know whether such a dose would relieve the pain of terminal cancer patients. If so, vitamin C might not only relieve pain, but serve to prolong life.

Vitamin C's potent antioxidant action is capable of removing carbon monoxide from hemoglobin when 12 to 50 grams are given intravenously within a short period of time. Such prompt treatment could prevent or reduce brain damage from lack of oxygen.

Vitamin C is the body's main protection against free radical damage within the brain. Therefore, there is an efficient pump mechanism that concentrates vitamin C within the brain to about one hundred times normal blood levels. An additional pump mechanism further concentrates the vitamin within nerve cells another hundred times. In times of cerebral anoxia, when free radicals increase a million-fold, vitamin C will minimize damage. Thus, keeping your levels of vitamin C high will reduce the risk of permanent central nervous system (brain and spinal cord) damage in case of accident or stroke. Since free radical damage occurs almost within minutes, vitamin C is more effective taken before an anoxic episode. Since cerebral ischemia can occur during anesthesia and surgery, this is another reason why patients undergoing surgery should be premedicated with vitamin C.

Doctors at Georgetown University Medical Center have proven that 2 grams of vitamin C daily will prevent many of the complications of steroid therapy. The effect was so good that it might be said that any long-term steroid therapy should include vitamin C to protect the patient from complications.

Vitamin C is required for the synthesis of bile from cholesterol, and increases the solubility of cholesterol in bile. This, plus its antioxidant properties, results in a reduction in blood cholesterol with as little as 200 milligrams of the vitamin daily over several months. Choline will increase this benefit.

Vitamin C is also a chelating agent, albeit a weak one. A chelating agent is able to bind itself to an atom and make it harmless and soluble. This chelating activity of vitamin C has been used to remove toxic lead, cadmium, and mercury poisoning. This benefit of vitamin C is far from academic, since toxic heavy metal loads have resulted in sperm counts that are only 20 percent of normal in one study at Florida State University, and fully 23 percent of those tested (132 students) could be considered sterile. Not all of this is the effect of toxic heavy metals, but is thought to be the combined effect of heavy metals and industrial chemicals. Persons with heavy metal poisoning should seriously consider taking several thousand milligrams of vitamin C daily. A periodic hair analysis is recommended.

By all means, I strongly recommend taking a minimum of 250 milligrams per day, and increasing that to as much as 10 grams per day in divided doses at the first sign of illness or during stress. Since body stores are increased through ingestion of 500 milligrams per day, that is the most logical daily dose. If this is taken either in divided doses or as a sustained release tablet it will be more effective. As a daily supplement, I prefer vitamin C buffered with trace elements and mixed with bioflavinoids.

Vitamin P, Bioflavinoids

The sources of bioflavinoids are the same as for vitamin C, except that the bioflavinoids are found in the pulp and peelings of citrus and peppers, rather than in the juice. The white pulp and core are especially rich in this vitamin.

Vitamin C never occurs alone in nature, but always is found with vitamin P. Because vitamin P deficiencies have been so hard to prove, this vitamin complex usually goes by the name bioflavinoids, at least in the United States where the FDA refuses to acknowledge the evidence. Nevertheless, there was a time shortly after the end of World War II when vitamin P deficiencies were demonstrable in Europe. In spite of official protests, there is ample clinical and scientific evidence that the bioflavinoids are active in human nutrition, and function to strengthen blood vessels and reduce capillary permeability. Capillaries have to leak somewhat, of course, to allow nutrients to get to the cells. But when capillaries are too leaky, edema results. Edema is the medical name for swelling due to excess fluid in the tissues of the body. In most cases, the edema is relatively harmless; but in all cases edema will reduce oxygen levels for the cells, and thus delay healing. A reduction in oxygen levels will increase the production of free radicals, with all its resultant pathology. If edema is severe, it can result in the death of tissue with possible loss of skin, or even a foot or hand. This is particularly common with diabetics.

Sometimes edema occurs in critical places, such as the eye. When edema develops in the back of the eye, astigmatism and poor central vision may result. If it persists for many weeks, loss of vision may be permament. Some years ago, I began using vitamin C and bioflavinoids in treatment of such diseases, with results at least equal to the best alternate therapies available, but without the serious risks nor expense. Generally, I will use bioflavinoids plus other vitamins for at least two weeks before going to more risky and expensive methods of treatment.

Within the past year a patient came to me after having successful cataract surgery which was later complicated by macular edema. When I saw her, the edema and blindness had persisted for about ten years. I referred her to a retina specialist to see whether laser treatment would be beneficial. His report was that no benefit was possible. Having nothing else to offer, I began her on vitamin E, vitamin C, bioflavinoids, plus large doses of multivitamins and minerals. Within five months her vision began to improve, and by nine months she could see well enough to pass a driver's examination. Too often novices in nutritional therapy become discouraged when no improvement develops within a few days. It generally took years of chronic malnutrition to produce the disease, and it will generally take months to years to reverse the damage. Some of my patients were still improving two years after treatment was begun. Some diseases show no measureable improvement for over three months. Others show improvement in just a few days. If the disease is acute, expect more rapid improvement with adequate doses of vitamins. Chronic diseases take longer. Unfortunately, advertising and our instant gratification culture has resulted in a population unwilling to wait for anything. This attitude makes the effective use of nutritional therapy very difficult.

Bioflavinoids have been proven to prevent clumping of red blood cells, and to be more potent than heparin in preventing certain types of thrombosis (blood clots). Prevention of clumping of blood cells would be a major safety factor for those exposed to possible frostbite, and for reducing the extent of injury from burns and crushing injuries. This could be of major benefit to those patients undergoing surgery, especially surgery that might compromise circulation, or workers or soldiers who risk serious injury. Much of the death of cells and tissue damage from burns, frostbite, and trauma occurs because capillaries leak fluid into the surrounding tissue so that oxygen cannot get to the cells; and because the abnormal situation causes blood cells to clump together so that they will not flow through the small capillaries. Bioflavinoids are a natural means of possibly reducing or even preventing injury under these circumstances. Needless to say, the bioflavinoids would be most effective if present before the injury.

This might be an appropriate place to diverge and consider what vitamins would most prevent serious permanent damage after an injury, whether by heat, cold, or physical trauma. Persons at risk of injury are advised to be prepared. Bioflavinoids and vitamin E would be effective in preventing clumping of cells inside injured blood vessels, and thereby would tend to prevent thrombosis. Neither vitamin prevents clotting outside blood vessels, so there would be no increased risk of hemorrhage such as occurs with other potent anti-clotting drugs. Additionally, vitamin C and bioflavinoids strengthen capillary walls to help them resist injury, and to prevent leakage of fluid into the surrounding tissue. Whatever leakage does occur as a result of the injury, the damage to the surrounding cells would be reduced by the oxygen sparing effects of vitamin E, vitamin C, and selenium. Incidentally, one of

123

the tests for vitamin C deficiency has been to place a tourniquet around the arm for several minutes, and count the number of hemorrhages that occur. A person deficient in vitamin C and bioflavinoids will bruise easily. Finally, aspirin, two tablets per week, will also reduce the risk of thrombosis and its complications. In the game of life you should play with a stacked deck. The entire spectrum of anti-free radical nutrients (beta carotene, vitamin E, vitamin C, selenium, riboflavin, and niacin) will greatly reduce the damage from injury, whether from burns, crushing, or laceration. Obviously, they will be more effective taken before the injury.

For optimum benefit, bioflavinoids should be taken with vitamin C, as they are found in nature. A sustained release product will eliminate the need for frequent consumption, and reduce the total quantity needed. Some individuals are intolerant of sustained release products, however.

Quercitin, one of the bioflavinoids, has now been proven to prevent a particular type of diabetic cataract that develops during periods of prolonged elevation of blood glucose levels. This diabetic cataract is formed when glucose which has entered the lens of the eye becomes converted to a more complex sugar molecule which cannot pass out of the lens membrane. This causes extra water to flow into the lens, producing edema (swelling) and cloudiness. Quercitin blocks the conversion of glucose to this more complex sugar (aldose), and thereby prevents the formation of the diabetic cataract.

My personal experience is that increasing the amount of vitamin C and P taken immediately at the first sign of illness will abort the illness. Generally, I will take about 1 gram of vitamin C every four hours, or if using a sustained release product this can be reduced to about 500 milligrams per dose. Using this program, I have rarely been ill for more than twelve hours, and then usually only inconvenienced. Good nutrition would have a greater impact on the cost of health care than anything we could possibly do other than perhaps stopping smoking or increasing our physical activities.

The Fat-Soluble Vitamins
Vitamins A, D, E, and K

The fat soluble vitamins are stored in the body, and toxic doses are possible. For vitamin A, doses of as high as 50,000 units daily are safe for many months, and 25,000 units of vitamin A is safe indefinitely.

Synthetic vitamin D is very apt to produce toxic symptoms, but the natural vitamin is certainly safe at 800 units daily, and probably always safe at 1000 units daily. Toxic reactions to natural vitamin D have not been recorded. However, vitamin D is added to so many processed foods that we in the U.S. are getting much more than we need without taking any supplemental vitamin D. In fact we are already getting toxic levels of supplemental vitamin D, an average of 3000 units per day!

Vitamin E is virtually non-toxic. Diarrhea has occurred with a single 6000 IU dose, and one person developed severe itching after taking 85,000 IU daily for over six months. The amazing thing is how he could afford such a dose.

Vitamin K is non-toxic except in those persons taking anti-coagulants, such as coumadin. It is synthesized in the intestine and supplementation is generally not necessary.

Vitamin A

RECOMMENDED DAILY ALLOWANCES (USDA):

Infants	1,500 IU
Children	2,500 IU
Adults	5,000 IU
Pregnant or lactating	8,000 IU

MAJOR SOURCES:
- Green and yellow vegetables (as beta carotene)
- Eggs
- Fish liver oils
- Liver
- Butter

Vitamin A from vegetable sources (beta carotene) is water soluble, and can never be toxic. The body converts these to the fat soluble retinol for storage only as needed. However, diabetics cannot generally make this conversion, and require dietary retinol, the fat soluble form of vitamin A.

Vitamin A from animal products (liver, eggs, butter, fish liver oils) are fat soluble. It is possible to take toxic amounts of this form of vitamin A. However, 25,000 IU is safe indefinitely. 100,000 IU daily may produce toxic effects after six or more months.

MAJOR BENEFITS:
Protein synthesis
Bone growth
Healthy skin
Sexual functions
Antioxidant/anticancer role (beta carotene)

DEFICIENCY SIGNS:
Night blindness
Reduced color vision
Dry eyes
Eye ulcers and infections
Glaucoma
Hard, dry, itching skin

Vitamin A was first called the "growth vitamin," and for good reason. Growth of animals deprived of vitamin A is greatly stunted. Almost everyone is aware that vitamin A is good for vision. Most are not aware that without zinc, vitamin A cannot be moved from the liver to the eyes where it can be used. Additionally, vitamin E is required for vitamin A to function properly in the eye, and protects vitamin A from oxidation into toxic metabolic by-products. Whether vitamin E works with vitamin A in its other roles is currently unknown.

Within the past two years, I have examined dozens of children with a deterioration of color vision, stereopsis, and vision, who rapidly responded to vitamin A therapy. Most of these children also had lost much of their ability to focus at near. Recovery with nutritional therapy was within six weeks. I have also had many patients whose glaucoma responded to vitamin A and manganese supplements over a six-month period of time.

Most of our vitamin A comes from vegetable sources, and is converted to retinol (the fat soluble form) as it is needed. The beta carotenes, which give yellow vegetables their color, are water soluble and non-toxic. There is strong scientific evidence that the beta carotenes provide considerable protection against cancer, the result of their ability to neutralize singlet oxygen, the most reactive free radical. Unfortunately, diabetics cannot convert beta carotene to retinol, so that diabetics must take their vitamin A in the fat soluble form. Fish liver oil, eggs, and liver are the best sources of retinol.

In 1955, the USDA concluded that in spite of the fact that 60 percent of the population ate a "good" diet, vitamin A was the principle nutrient lacking in the diet. Since 1955, concern over obesity and cholesterol have reduced the ingestion of eggs. Liver has never been a popular food item, and almost no one takes fish liver oils. The shift to processed foods has further reduced the consumption of green and yellow vegetables. As a result, we should expect that vitamin A deficiencies are very common today.

A panel investigating human nutrition in the U.S. in 1968 concluded that 40 percent of all Americans are deficient in vitamin A, and that as a result as many as 46 percent of children in some states suffer stunted growth. The human liver can easily store 500,000 IU of vitamin A, a three-month's supply if we are to believe the USDA's RDA. Nevertheless, Canadian authorities performed autopsies on 100 subjects to determine vitamin A stores, and found that fully 10 percent had zero reserves! An additional 21 percent had virtually no reserves. Add to that the fact that zinc is necessary to use vitamin A, and the fact that more recent studies reveal that 85 percent of the American population is zinc deficient, and it is easy to understand why is it not only possible, but likely, that vitamin A deficiencies are common.

USDA statistics show that the average American today annually consumes 31 fewer pounds of fresh fruit, and 20 fewer pounds of fresh vegetables than in 1950. Thus the average diet that left 40 percent deficient in 1955 now provides 225,000 IU less vitamin A today. This is fifty-one days' supply of the RDA. If we had shifted our diet to liver and eggs, there would not have been a problem. The opposite has occurred: we have shifted our diet away from *every* good source of vitamin A.

Additionally, vitamin A is destroyed by many products of modern society. Air pollution in most forms destroys vitamin A. So do the nitrites added to processed meats such as bologna, hot dogs, and hams. The nitrites used in commercial fertilizers destroys much of the vitamin A activity in fresh vegetables; and so does cooking, which is necessary in the canning process.

How much vitamin A is necessary for good health? A lot will depend upon your past diet, your exposure to pollutants including smoking, and your age. If you have neglected fresh green and yellow vegetables, and are not a lover of liver nor eggs, then assume that your vitamin A reserves are nil. If you are diabetic, then you cannot convert beta carotene to retinol, and you must ignore vegetables as a source of vitamin A. That is not to say that you should not be eating vegetables; but rather, don't consider them as a source of vitamin A. You will still need to consume foods rich in beta carotene to protect yourself against free radical pathology. If you are zinc deficient, and 85 percent of the population is, then whatever vitamin A you do have stored is doing you precious little good. If these statements apply to you, consider that you could take up to about 500,000 units within a week's time without problems. After that, you can safely ingest at least 20,000 IU of retinol daily, and up to 100,000 IU of beta carotene daily. The best way to get your beta carotene is from foods rich in that pro-vitamin: yellow fruit and vegetables (two servings daily), and dark green leafy vegetables (especially broccoli and spinach).

In summary, there is strong evidence that the average American's diet is vitamin A deficient. Also, the ravages of modern society have greatly increased the need for this vitamin, and reduced its supply in the diet. The results of this deficiency are poor growth, eye diseases, reduced resistance to infection, and an increased incidence of cancer. By all means, shift your diet toward more fresh green and yellow vegetables, and supplement your diet with at least 5,000 IU of retinol daily. Beta carotene can be obtained by two or more servings of green or yellow vegetables daily, broccoli being an especially good source. Amazingly, one ounce of beef liver contains 15,000 IU of retinol. Obviously, a serving of just over four ounces of beef liver every two weeks will supply all your requirements of retinol. A single egg supplies about 300 IU of the vitamin, and supplies even more if it is cooked in butter.

Vitamin D

Vitamin D is a group of related compounds, similar to cholesterol. The skin can make vitamin D when exposed to sunshine. There is ample evidence that the synthetic forms of vitamin D are the most toxic of this group. Although vitamin D was used extensively before 1942, toxic reactions did not occur until after synthetic forms were introduced. The toxic effects in infants proven to be due to vitamin D all developed with the use of the synthetic D2 vitamin. There are no documented toxic reactions with the natural forms of vitamin D. However, so many foods have supplemental synthetic vitamin D added that Americans are getting over seven times our minimal needs without supplementation. Vitamin D toxicity is occurring as a result. Unless you have a proven deficiency in this vitamin you should avoid supplementation.

The D vitamins are stored in the liver. Sunshine has been our principle source of this vitamin, since one square centimeter of skin can synthesize 18 IU of vitamin D in three hours of exposure to full sunshine. Translated into useful terms, two minutes on the beach will provide your daily quota of vitamin D. This is reduced by a tan or even more so in blacks, since melanin serves to screen out the ultraviolet light which catalyses the synthesis. Quite obviously, our ancestors many centuries ago were synthesizing many times the RDA of natural vitamin D. Smog will reduce the amount of ultraviolet light significantly. In fact, vitamin D deficiency was unknown until after the Industrial Revolution and its pollution. Vitamin D deficiency rarely occurs in the far northern oceana countries because their diet contains a healthy sampling of marine fish with their high vitamin D content. (Isn't it amazing that our Creator would have provided that those who live too far north to get ample vitamin D from sunshine would get it from the fish that frequent the northern oceans?)

Do vitamin D deficiencies actually occur? Studies have shown that vitamin D levels in the blood are highest in September, and lowest in December. Interestingly, osteomalacia, a disease of weakened bones, occurs more frequently in early spring when the toll of poor calcium absorption would be expected to peak. Since vitamin D is necessary for calcium to be absorbed, it is reasonable to assume that the high incidence of osteoporosis present in the elderly is at least in part due to vitamin D deficiency. However, the elderly tend to spend less time in the sunlight, and also have diets that are generally deficient in all nutrients. The frequency at which elderly persons break bones is well known, and this is a direct result of calcium and vitamin D deficiency. Without vitamin D, of course, you can eat calcium supplements until your bowels turn to concrete and your bones will still be soft and brittle. I again wish to emphasize that vitamin D toxicity is a greater problem in most people between adolescence and perhaps age 60 or older.

It may come as a surprise, but your bones are not chunks of stone. Bone is a living organ which is constantly being restructured for maximum strength with minimum weight. When you exercise, stresses are placed on the bones, and each bone will change its shape and internal structure over a period of several weeks to meet its new demands. This is why a pathologist can frequently determine the occupation of a person by examining the bones. Each job stresses different bones. Likewise, when you begin a new type of work, several weeks are required for the bones to adjust. Without vitamin D (and vitamins A, C, and calcium), this remolding process cannot occur. Bone design is an engineer's dream. Bone is a living structure, and is constantly changing. When your bones do not get enough vitamin D and minerals, they complain with pain and fractures.

Vitamin D deficiency may have effects that are totally unexpected. For example, hearing depends upon the integrity of three tiny bones in the middle ear, and upon the flexibility of their interconnections (joints). A recent study in England (where vitamin D supplementation is not so severe) cited in the *Journal of the American Medical Association* (November, 1983) demonstrated an association of hearing loss with vitamin D deficiency. Interestingly, the loss was in the higher frequencies usually associated with noise trauma. Further studies are being done to clarify the association, which seems logical once you consider the role of these three tiny bones.

There are other studies which suggest that vitamin D supplementation of foods is so widespread that we might be getting seven times or more of our RDA without knowing it. The safest course would be to have a vitamin D assay run before taking supplemental vitamin D. However, since there have been no recognized toxic effects with natural vitamin D, an alternate safe approach might be to use only supplements which use natural vitamin D, and limit that to 800 IU per day unless a deficiency has been proven. Getting your vitamin D from exposure to sunshine would be the most natural way to obtain the vitamin.

Vitamin E

RECOMMENDED DAILY ALLOWANCES:

Infant	5 IU
Children	10 IU
All others	30 IU

(See paragraph two below.)

MAJOR SOURCES:
Green leafy vegetables
Whole grains (fresh only)
Safflower oil (fresh)

What germ (fresh)

Peanuts

MAJOR BENEFITS:

Dissolves fibrin (blood clots)

Antioxidant

Protects red blood cells from lysis

Reduces thrombin formation

Protects against cancer and aging due to oxidation

(*All* of the above are the result of neutralization of free radicals.)

Vitamin E's primary, and perhaps only, function is to intercept and neutralize free radicals. In the process, vitamin E is oxidized to tocoperol quinone, and is regenerated to vitamin E by the action of vitamin C. However, even though vitamin E is effective in scavenging free radicals, it is more effective when the diet supplies adequate selenium. The selenium ion is also effective as a free radical scavenger, and also acts as part of the enzyme glutathione peroxidase (which is part of a chain of reactions that recycles nutrients used in our battle against free radicals.) Since selenium and vitamin C deficiencies are now known to be common, it is no wonder that studies using minimal doses of vitamin E have shown no effect. Vitamin E works quickly to neutralize free radicals, but it may take six weeks to a year to get the maximum benefits of vitamin E therapy because one the ongoing pathology is stopped, repairs must be begun, and that takes time. Only in the case of inflammatory diseases, and acute burns and injury does the vitamin seem to have an immediate effect.

The officially accepted RDA for vitamin E was calculated by Dr. M. K. Horwitt, who later discovered an error in his calculations, and who now recommends about 800 IU as safe. The recommended daily allowance by the new calculations is ten to twenty times the official recommendation. In any case, the average American diet supplies less than 10 IU daily, as determined by the National Institutes of Health. Anyone who says vitamin E supplementation is not necessary is simply ignorant. However, now that the role of vitamin C in recycling vitamin E has been established, new calculations will have to be done while supplying the nutrients used in the regenerative metabolic pathways. In the meantime, I believe a minimum of 400 IU daily is needed to meet all the demands placed upon this essential vitamin by our environment and diet.

Vitamin E is indirectly destroyed by inorganic iron, which is a potent catalyst of free radicals which this vitamin must neutralize. Excess copper also has the same effect. Chlorine, used to purify water in most cities, is a powerful oxidant and instantly destroys vitamin E. This is especially interesting because studies in the early 1950s have proven that chlorine in drinking water produces atherosclerosis, at least in chickens. I have absolutely no doubt that chlorinated water does the same to humans. Other studies have shown that vitamin E will prevent and even reverse atherosclerosis. The relationship should be obvious. Vitamin E is also destroyed by milling and bleaching flour, and is not added to so-called enriched flour. It is also destroyed by prolonged cooking, and the canning process. Canned vegetables are almost devoid of vitamin E. Only fresh vegetables eaten raw or with minimal cooking have significant amounts of this vitamin. Vegetable oils are touted to be excellent sources of vitamin E, and they are: but only if the oil has been cold pressed in an inert gas atmosphere, a prohibitively expensive process which is never done commercially. Unfortunately, vegetable oils are susceptible to oxidation and production of carcinogenic free radicals, and require additional vitamin E to prevent this. Only cottonseed oil contains enough vitamin E to protect it from oxidation: use of other oils increases the need for vitamin E. Soybean oil, the most commonly used, is especially low in vitamin E. Even worse, the current high market value for vitamin E has made it profitable for industry to remove the vitamin E from oils before marketing the oil. In short, vegetable oils are no longer a good source of vitamin E. (Olive oil is more saturated and less likely to be rancid.)

This past week it was announced that it is thought that the increase in incidence of stomach cancer in the U.S. is the result of the reuse of cooking oils in fast food restaurants. The protective vitamin E is destroyed with the initial use of cooking oil, after which the oil is quickly oxidized to produce toxic compounds. Synthetic antioxidants such as BHA or BHT could be added to prevent this oxidation.

Vitamin E is consumed by physical activity. Studies in Russia have shown that training athletes need at least 75 milligrams (units) of vitamin E per hour of hard work. A man doing heavy manual labor should be taking at least 600 IU daily. In recent years, all winners of the Olympics have been on vitamin E supplements both during training and competition. Careful studies have confirmed this benefit.

Vitamin E will pass through the skin. When applied to the skin immediately after a burn, the damage is greatly reduced. This has been confirmed by applying vitamin E to one side of the back of a man exposed to excessive sunlight. The side treated with vitamin E usually will not become red nor peel. Vitamin E acts to stabilize the cell walls by its prevention of free radical damage so that the cells do not die. Edema and inflammation are thus prevented.

Vitamin E taken before exposure to sunlight will also reduce sunburn. I have taken 1000 IU of vitamin E daily before working under clear spring skies for two full twelve-hour days, without other protection, without a prior tan, and without burning. My two sons were also similarly exposed, and were not burned. Without the protection of vitamin E we would have peeled like a snake. Dr. Cranton points out that beta carotene is even more effective against sunburn, a thesis supported by the experience of Durk Pearson and Sandy Shaw. Since sunlight burns by the production of free radicals, keeping yourself primed with those nutrients mentioned in an earlier chapter on defense against free radical damage will help prevent sunburn. Note, however, that there will be a limit to your indiscretion.

Vitamin E does not pass the placental barrier, however, and every child is born deficient in vitamin E. The unborn child therefore depends upon selenium and beta carotene to protect it against free radical pathology. If the nursing mother is taking sufficient vitamin E, then the infant will get his supply quickly enough, since Vitamin E is concentrated in human milk. That is, unless the mother cleans her nipples before nursing, thereby removing the fat soluble vitamins excreted there for the infant. For the infant's sake, any nursing mother should take supplementary vitamin E. Anemia and jaundice due to vitamin E deficiency has been confirmed in infants. More recent infant formulas have sufficient vitamin E added to prevent anemia, but this is of no value to an infant who is breast fed, and whose mother is deficient in vitamin E. Cow's milk does not contain vitamin E.

Vitamin E promotes healing. Patients who have had surgery heal faster with smaller scars when vitamin E is used. My cataract patients begin recovering vision after cataract surgery in just a few days compared to the several weeks required before I began using 1200 IU of vitamin E before and after surgery.

Since vitamin E dissolves fibrin and reduces thrombin production, it acts to prevent clotting of blood within a blood vessel. There is clear evidence that vitamin E, taken in sufficient quantity, will reduce the incidence of thrombosis and strokes, and further that vitamin E will speed the healing of thrombophlebitis.

Sufficient quantity means at least 1200 IU daily. This effect of vitamin E is due again to its ability to neutralize free radicals. A high density of free radicals will cause blood to clot.

The many facets of vitamin E are explained by several of the effects of this versatile vitamin: vitamin E reduces the need for oxygen; at the same time, vitamin E also seems to encourage the growth of new small blood vessels into active muscles. Vitamin E reduces the need for steroids in inflammation, a fact emphasized in the Jackson Memorial Lecture at the 1983 annual American Academy of Ophthalmology meeting in Chicago. By stabilizing cell membranes, vitamin E reduces capillary leakage so that fluid stays within the blood vessels, where it belongs. And, perhaps most importantly, the ability of vitamin E to neutralize free radicals makes it essential in prevention of the various types of free radical pathology.

In spite of official protests, careful double-blind studies have proven that vitamin E does improve cardiac function, and allows more blood to flow within atherosclerotic vessels. It has also been proven that vitamin E increases the distance a person can walk without leg cramps, and that angina (heart pains due to poor circulation) is both less frequent and less severe. Canadian statistics show that a person taking 800 IU of vitamin E daily is only half as likely to have a heart attack; and, if he has his attack, he is twice as likely to leave the hospital alive. Put another way, a man is four times as likely to be alive a year from now if he is daily taking 800 IU of vitamin E. More recent studies in Finland showed that only four persons out of a random sampling of 2400 persons over 60 years of age who had also taken at least 400 IU of vitamin E daily for over ten years had any evidence of cardiovascular disease. The expected incidence would have been 800 victims, two hundred times as many. Such is the devastation of free radical pathology.

My experience has confirmed that fully nine out of ten persons with reduced visual acuity without obvious cause have improved vision upon treatment with vitamin E. Several patients whose vision had deteriorated to bare hand movement have recovered to useful vision, including being able to read without special aids. Studies released by the National Institutes of Health in September, 1983, have proven that vitamin E is essential for vision, seemingly playing a role in protecting vitamin A from toxic oxidation. This confirmation of my observations is comforting, to say the least. I cannot claim uniqueness in this discovery, because this benefit has been noted by other physicians, the first being Dr. George Dowd. Most certainly, I was not taught this effect at any time during my residency training.

Since vitamin E reduces the need for oxygen, those diseases which are characterized by oxygen deficiency should be treated with vitamin E supplements. These diseases include diabetes mellitus, thrombosis, stroke, macular diseases of the eye, and all vascular diseases including cardiovascular disease and poor circulation. Apparently, persons who have rheumatic heart disease are very sensitive to vitamin E, and treatment should be cautious. Whether this risk is due to concurrent selenium or magnesium deficiency is unknown.

Vitamin E's antioxidant effect makes it one of the vitamins effective in preventing cancer. It also makes it effective in slowing aging due to free radical formation and cross linkage of body proteins. Not that vitamin E can restore a man to the condition he was in during his 20s, but it certainly appears to help hold the line.

Do yourself a favor and supplement your diet with at least 400 IU of vitamin E plus selenium daily. Also shift your diet to include more raw and fresh vegetables, especially cabbage, spinach, asparagus, and broccoli. Incidentally, it is the core of the cabbage head which contains the vitamin. Whole grain and wheat germ are also good sources, but only if they are fresh. Vegetable oils are not a good source because they also increase your need for vitamin E.

Certain events require additional vitamin E. Take more before doing strenuous work, and before and after prolonged exposure to the sun. Persons exposed to ionizing radiation (such as radiologists and radiation technicians) should increase their consumption of the vitamin, as should anyone exposed to pollution, including smoking. If you drink chlorinated city water, then take steps to eliminate it from your drinking water and also increase your intake of vitamin E. Chlorine can be eliminated by letting water stand in an open jar overnight, as in a refrigerator, boiling drinking water briefly, or by using special filters sold for that purpose.

Incidentally, if you start taking vitamin E, do not expect to see instant changes. Generally improvement will occur over a period of at least six weeks. It also takes several days without the vitamin supplement before any decrease in vitality is noticed. The only exceptions are those involving acute inflammation, which respond rapidly.

XVIII.
The Stagehands of Life

MAJOR SOURCES:
  Whole grain cereals
  Brewer's yeast
  Liver
  Kidney
  Milk
  Eggs
  Peanuts
  Lentils

THE VITAMINS AND THEIR MAJOR METABOLIC FUNCTIONS:

Thiamine	Carbohydrate
Riboflavin	Carbohydrate and protein
	Antioxidant
Niacin	Carbohydrate and protein
	Critical to all energy production
	Antioxidant
Pyridoxine	Carbohydrate, fat, and protein
Pantothenic acid	Carbohydrate, fat, and protein
Folice acid	DNA, RNA, cell reproduction
Cyanocobalamine	DNA, RNA, protein
Biotin	Many functions
Choline	Nerve function
Inositol	Nerve, function, Cholesterol control,
	and Cancer inhibition

The B vitamins are a group of water soluble vitamins that are intimately involved in all metabolic activities of the body. Without these vitamins daily in our diet, we cannot live in optimum health.

The B vitamins do not work alone, but in cooperation with each other and other vitamins and minerals. Therefore it is important that your vitamin intake be balanced so that metabolic processes are not forced in a direction not desired. The B vitamins especially act as catalysts to bring special molecules together for the production of energy, protein, or other necessary purposes.

Some of these vitamins are not true vitamins in that we can manufacture them to a limited degree within our own bodies. Nevertheless, that manufacturing is limited by other nutrients which cannot produce internally, but must supply in the diet. By supplying these essential non-vitamins in the diet, the body's need for the true vitamins and amino acids is reduced. For the ones listed, it has been clearly shown that their addition to the diet results in improvement in health. For that reason, I will treat them as vitamins.

Being water soluble, these vitamins are not stored, and must be in the daily diet. since they are involved in different aspects of metabolism, the actual amount of each will vary with the diet and activities. For example, a diet rich in carbohydrates requires more thiamine to use that food. Extra thiamine is also needed by a person who is physically active and burning more calories. An automobile will not run without fuel, but neither will it run without some means of burning that fuel. The B vitamins are the spark plugs in our energy system.

Quite frankly, it is probable that there are yet undiscovered vitamins. Certainly, discoveries in nutrition are still being made. Only within the past few years have we discovered the importance of chromium, zinc, and selenium. And we still don't know exactly what these minerals do. It has taken three decades to unravel the complex problem of free radical pathology, and begin to tie the loose ends together. There is much more to be learned.

This is mentioned to emphasize the importance of using natural sources of vitamins and minerals whenever possible. It is likely that other unknown vitamins will be found together in nature, so that you will be getting the essentials without fail. Synthetic vitamins, although identical to the natural ones in most cases, cannot supply vitamins and minerals that are not known. The most economical approach will be a combination of natural and synthetic vitamins.

Thiamine, Vitamin B1

RECOMMENDED DAILY ALLOWANCES:

Infants	0.5 mg.
Children	0.7 mg.
Adults	1.7 mg.

MAJOR SOURCES:
    Whole grain cereals

Liver
Pork
Fresh green vegetables
Potatoes
Beans   ·
Brewer's yeast
MAJOR BENEFITS:
   Cell oxidation
   Growth
   Appetite enhancement
   Carbohydrate metabolism
   Nerve function
   Heart health
   The primary function of thiamine is the oxidation of glucose in the production of energy. Glucose is the main form of fuel used throughout the body, and it is the only fuel that the brain and nervous system can use. (Dextrose is another name for glucose, the major ingredient in corn syrup.) That is why thiamine deficiency affects the nervous system so quickly. The muscles and heart can use other fuels, but glucose is the primary fuel, and the alternate fuels are the by-products of glucose metabolism.

   Beriberi is a fatal disease of muscle weakness, heart failure, and eventual paralysis and death. It first became apparent when civilized polished white rice was substituted for unpolished brown rice. Most of the vitamins in rice are in the bran outer coating of the grain. The same is true for other cereal grains, in which the nutritious coating is usually milled off. This is another example of how God has provided with the grain the vitamins necessary for our use of the nutrition in the grain.

   After it was discovered that thiamine was needed to use the food value of the rice, millers began to add thiamine back to their milled rice and other grains. However, they added only 20 percent of the thiamine they had removed. Furthermore, the list of food sources of thiamine makes it obvious that many are no longer consumed in quantity.

   Additionally, thiamine is destroyed by high heat, and is lost if water used in cooking is thrown away. Since thiamine is water soluble, it cannot be stored appreciably, and should be included in the daily diet.

   The need for thiamine varies with the diet, and with activity. A physically active man requires approximately twice as much as an inactive man. A diet high in carbohydrates requires more thiamine. Alcohol not only requires thiamine for detoxification, but reduces absorption, and substitues for foods that may have had thiamine.

The full spectrum of nutrients in bran is unknown, and became known only through deficiency and the inquiring mind of someone with skills and money to pursue research. It is unlikely that all the nutrients in bran will be discovered, and therefore no synthetic substitute will have all the nutrients available in the natural sources. For these and other reasons, plan to get the extra vitamins you need from natural sources insofar as possible.

Even with "enrichment" of breads and rice, only a few of the known nutrients in bran are replaced, and those replaced are insufficient. During milling of flour, twenty-six vitamins and minerals proven to be essential for life are removed. "Enrichment" partially replaces three of the vitamins plus iron. A partial list of the nutrients *removed* includes:

77 percent of vitamin B1
80 percent of vitamin B2
81 percent of vitamin B3
50 percent of pantothenic acid
72 percent of vitamin B6
86 percent of vitamin E
27 percent of the protein
60 percent of the calcium
76 percent of the iron
85 percent of the magnesium
78 percent of the zinc

And they have the audacity to call it enriched! Additionally, many of the popular foods are not enriched at all. There is ample evidence that most of our population is subsisting at the edge of thiamine deficiency.

The early signs of thiamine deficiency are fatigue, loss of appetite, irritability, and poor memory. As deficiency becomes more severe there will be tingling of the hands and toes, bursts of emotion, vague pains, and cardiac insufficiency. These are all too common in all of us. My personal experience is that I have rarely been tired since beginning on vitamin B supplements.

Several studies have shown that heart disease and complaints are more common in those who eat a diet high in processed carbohydrates, especially sugar. The incidence of heart disease almost parallels the lack of thiamine in the diet. What else should we expect?

Pathological evidence confirms that although thiamine will reverse much of the disability due to its deficiency, permanent damage does occur to both the nerves and heart muscle. The risk of permanent damage is ample reason to supplement your diet daily with thiamine.

In studies done in the U.S. and Switzerland, it has been proven that thiamine given to children increases mental performance by as much as 32 percent. Roy Haupt, my eighth-grade teacher, told me of a study he did in which he got children to record their daily diet. The records were coded for objectivity. After a year, the code was broken. The clear finding was that scholastic performance was directly related to nutrition; and more specifically, to the quality of breakfast eaten. The data was given to the school board, and has been ignored. A similar study was done with students in the poorest section of Louisiana, where scholastic performance was the lowest in the state. After one year of nutritional supplementation, the students were performing near the top of their class. As it is said in computer jargon: garbage in, garbage out.

Riboflavin, Vitamin B2

RECOMMENDED DAILY ALLOWANCES:

Infants	0.6 mg.
Children	0.8 mg.
Adults	1.7 mg.
Lactating	2.0 mg.

MAJOR SOURCES:
  Brewer's yeast
  Beef kidney
  Beef liver
  Wheat germ
  Green leafy vegetables
  Peas
  Lima beans

MAJOR BENEFITS:
  Protein metabolism
  Fat metabolism
  Liver, skin, eye function
  Involvement in free radical protection

Riboflavin is the yellow vitamin. It also has a distinctive odor. In generous quantities, it is said to discourage mosquitoes from biting, so this vitamin is popular with campers.

Riboflavin is necessary for fat metabolism. When riboflavin and tryptophan (an essential amino acid) are both available, the body can produce niacin, another B vitamin. Niacin, in turn, is important in recycling riboflavin in the metabolic chain involved in free radical neutralization. Folic acid, another B vitamin, cannot be used without ample riboflavin on board. New tissue cannot be formed, nor damaged tissue repaired, without riboflavin. As with all vitamins, it is essential for life.

Deficiencies produce most commonly lesions in the mucous membranes, those wet tissues of the body. These include the eyes, tongue, lips, and skin. Anemia can result since the body cannot use folic acid without riboflavin.

Deficiencies can exist without obvious signs. In one study a group of volunteers was put on a riboflavin deficient diet. Personality tests were given before and after the experiment. Defects in personality were noted by the sixth week of deprivation. The defects noted include fatigue, poor appetite, nervousness, depression, and hysteria. Does this sound like someone you know?

A USDA study in 1965 concluded that only half of American households include the RDA of riboflavin in their diet. A glance at the list of food sources rich in riboflavin clearly shows that our diet today is even less likely to contain riboflavin than in 1965. During the past ten years consumption has shifted strongly away from basic foods to processed foods and junk foods empty of everything except calories. It is highly unlikely that your diet has sufficient riboflavin.

Fresh milk once was an excellent source of riboflavin. But milk is treated with ultraviolet light to increase its vitamin D content, and ultraviolet light destroys riboflavin. Further, milk today is delivered in clear containers, increasing the destruction of this vitamin. This may be why fresh milk is more beneficial to some people. Riboflavin is destroyed by heat (cooking), and also by alcohol. Canned vegetables therefore would have lost their riboflavin content. Many Southerners cook vegetables until they are soft, destroying whatever nutrition had been there. The Yankee way of barely cooking vegetables is clearly superior. Some riboflavin seems to be destroyed by the use of oral contraceptives. How many of the symptoms that come with the use of the pill are no more than vitamin deficiency?

Birth defects in animals commonly occur when the mother is fed a riboflavin deficient diet. The defects are similar to those which occurred with Thalidomide. Since many of the symptoms one would treat with Thalidomide (a tranquilizer) are symptoms of riboflavin deficiency, one cannot help but wonder whether the real problem was riboflavin deficiency made worse by Thalidomide. No studies on riboflavin deficiency and birth defects in humans have been done.

Since riboflavin is water soluble, it would be difficult to get too much. Excess of any single vitamin, however, may push metabolic reactions in undesired directions, with unpredictable results. Megadosages of individual vitamins is not generally recommended. If your urine develops a strong yellow color within an hour of taking riboflavin, you are getting enough for that day. Generally, except in special situations, nutritional therapy should be with all the vitamins and minerals, and should be from natural sources whenever possible. Putting a new horse on a two-horse sleigh does not help if the other horse is exhausted.

Niacin, Vitamin B3

RECOMMENDED DAILY ALLOWANCES:

Infants	8 mg.
Children	9 mg.
Adults	20 mg.
Lactating	20 mg.

MAJOR SOURCES:
Brewer's yeast
Beef kidney
Beef liver
Fish
Poultry
Soybeans
Wheat germ
Peanut butter

MAJOR BENEFITS:
Carbohydrate metabolism
Circulatory system
Recycles riboflavin

Niacin is unique in that it can be synthesized from tryptophan (an essential amino acid), with the aid of thiamine, pyridoxine, and riboflavin. This conversion is inefficient, however, and uses up valuable tryptophan. Don't depend upon making your own for health.

There are two forms of this vitamin: niacin (otherwise called vitamin B3 or nicotinic acid), and niacinamide. Niacin causes dilation of blood vessels and is effective in reducing blood cholesterol and blood pressure. Niacinamide is usually used when enriching foods. Niacin is used therapeutically to dilate blood vessels in an effort to improve circulation, and frequently causes headache when more than 50 milligrams is used. Niacinamide does not cause dilation of blood vessels, nor does it reduce blood cholesterol. When choosing a B-complex supplement, it is preferable to choose one with niacin rather than niacinamide, unless you prove sensitive to the niacin. Even better, take niacin to the limits of your tolerance (about 50 to 100 milligrams), and make the rest up in niacinamide.

A study by HEW in 1972 concluded that 13 percent of all persons over 60 had clinical signs of niacin deficiency. Additionally, about 9 percent of persons above the poverty level, and 6 percent of those under the poverty level had clinical evidence of niacin deficiency. If this many of our citizens show clinical signs of deficiency, how many are borderline deficient?

More interestingly, niacin deficiency causes mental disturbances almost identical to schizophenia. Many years ago, psychiatrists distinguished between the two by administering niacin. If the patient got well, they had pellagra (the disease caused by niacin deficiency). If not, they were assumed to be schizophrenic. The fact that niacin deficiencies can produce hallucinations and distortions of perception (how we see and hear things) brings up some interesting questions. How often is the paranoid behavior of many elderly nothing more than a manifestation of niacin deficiency? If the lack of good nutrition leads to schizophrenic behavior, what happens when an entire society is deficient because it cannot supply a proper diet, a problem common in the Third World and some Communist Bloc nations? The answers to these questions are more than academic.

Since niacin is necessary and used up during carbohydrate metabolism, our modern diet of processed foods rich in starch (as a thickener) and sugar should require more niacin. These processed foods are exactly those from which vitamins have been removed. A quick glance at the list of foods rich in niacin will confirm that except for peanut butter, the average diet today contains none of these foods.

Niacin deficiency will show up as weakness, fatigue, irritability, or insomnia. Mental illness in some cases may be niacin deficiencies. More severe deficiencies may cause fissures of the tongue, and dry, coarse skin.

Niacin is lost in cooking; and as with all of the B vitamins, alcohol is highly destructive. Niacin is not toxic. Doses in excess of 100 milligrams may produce discomfort due to dilation of blood vessels.

Pyridoxine, Vitamin B6

RECOMMENDED DAILY ALLOWANCES:

Infants	0.4 mg.
Children	0.7 mg.
Adults	2 mg.
Lactating	2.5 mg.

MAJOR SOURCES:
Brewer's yeast
Beef kidney
Beef liver
Fish
Poultry (White meat)
Soybeans
Wheat germ
Peanut butter
Bananas
Filberts
Buckwheat flour

MAJOR BENEFITS:
Protein metabolism
Carbohydrate metabolism
Fat metabolism
Enzyme activator
Hormone production and use
Insulin production
DNA and RNA
Potassium and iron metabolism

Pyridoxine is involved in so many metabolic systems that it is difficult to grasp exactly what it is doing. It is necessary for many of the other vitamins to function. Vitamin B6 also requires magnesium as a cofactor.

Pyridoxine is destroyed by processing. It is required in greater quantities in persons on a high protein diet. Although the official RDA is 2 milligrams, many persons have been proven to require up to ten times this amount. One study has shown that three out of four diets are deficient in this vitamin.

Many diseases have been shown to respond to this vitamin. Most notable are acne, tooth decay, and atherosclerosis. The latter may be due to the fact that B6 is required to make lecithin, which is known to dissolve cholesterol deposits. Seborrheic dermatitis often responds to large doses of B6 both orally and topically. Some diabetes have been shown to respond to pyridoxine treatment, which perhaps should have been expected since it is necessary for insulin synthesis. Hypertension and edema of pregnancy can be treated with very large doses of pyridoxine plus magnesium. Incidentally, leg cramps are not always due to calcium deficiency. It can be due to vitamin E, magnesium, or pyridoxine deficiency. Milk is deficient both in pyridoxine and magnesium. Pyridoxine deficiency in animals leads to cancer. As with all of the B vitamins, pyridoxine deficiency causes mental and nervous disturbances.

Women especially need additional pyridoxine during pregnancy and when taking birth control pills. Patients on steroids require up to 20 milligrams per day of vitamin B6. Diabetics have now been shown to need additional B6, as well as magnesium, chromium, vitamin E, bioflavinoids, and vitamin C. In fact, some diabetics will respond to pyridoxine and magnesium therapy just as to supplemental insulin. A study done some years ago revealed that many asthmatics have an apparent pyridoxine dependent disease, which responds over a period of many months to high doses of the vitamin.

The fact that deficiencies of this vitamin are common, plus the more common lack of magnesium in the diet, strongly indicate supplementation with calcium/magnesium tablets and B Complex. Supplemental magnesium should always be used with pyridoxine, otherwise a magnesium deficiency may develop. The reverse is also true. A study in the *New England Journal of Medicine* (August 26, 1983) establishes that persons taking high doses of pyridoxine may develop neurological symptoms. This should have been anticipated, since administration of pyridoxine without supplemental magnesium may result in a magnesium deficiency, and even a mild magnesium deficiency results in serious neurological symptoms. In view of the NEJM article, which is the first toxic effect reported for one of the water soluble vitamins, be aware that by taking any of the vitamins in mega-doses there is the possibility of forcing metabolic pathways in ways you would not wish them to go, with deleterious effects. This problem is usually avoided by broad spectrum supplementation. I believe that the toxic effects reported with pyridoxine were in fact due to induced magnesium deficiency. The toxic dose of pyridoxine was at least 2 grams daily, a thousand times the RDA.

It is foolish to use potent medications in a patient before attempting to correct basic nutritional deficiencies which prevent healing. Treatment of any disease starts with a nutritional history. If deficiencies are probable, then those should be corrected first in order that maximum healing can occur. Just as a house cannot be built without building materials, a body cannot heal itself without those elements necessary for healing. This is so obvious it should be beyond debate. The fact that a book such as this must be written is ample evidence that the obvious is frequently overlooked by those who should know better.

Vitamin B12

RECOMMENDED DAILY ALLOWANCES:

Infants	2 micrograms
Children	3 micrograms
Adults	6 micrograms
Pregnant	8 micrograms

MAJOR DIETARY SOURCES:
    Yeast
    Wheat germ
    Liver
    Milk
    Eggs
    Meat
    Cheese

MAJOR FUNCTIONS:
    Red blood cell formation
    Nerve function
    RNA and DNA synthesis
    Carbohydrate metabolism
    Necessary for growth and healing
    Necessary for fertility

Vitamin B12 is absolutely necessary for life, yet it is needed in such small quantities that a teaspoon could hold the daily ration for almost three years. Its functions are intimately tied in with folic acid, and both are necessary for the synthesis of DNA and RNA, the stuff of life itself. Cells cannot reproduce without new DNA and RNA being made, and without cell division there is no healing nor growth. RNA is also used by the brain to store information. This RNA function of B12 may be the reason that mental and psychiatric manifestations of B12 deficiency may precede anemia by years. The fact that vitamin B12 deficiency can be present for years before anemia appears, with resulting permanent nerve damage, is all the more reason for being aware of its possibility.

The vitamin is rather common in the diet, so why should a deficiency occur? This vitamin will not pass through the walls of the intestine unless it is first attached to another compound, called "intrinsic factor." Some persons, however, cannot produce intrinsic factor, and therefore they cannot use the vitamin B12 in their diet. Since the loss of intrinsic factor is more than likely to be over a period of time, and since the amount of B12 needed is very small, the development of vitamin B12 deficiency is apt to be insidious. The anemia that develops will not respond to any dietary approach, and so was named pernicious anemia. Once it was discovered that the vitamin could be given by injection the cursed anemia was cured.

Obviously, if you have intrinsic factor, you cannot have a vitamin B12 deficiency. This, plus the fact that the vitamin is water soluble, gives us an easy way to diagnose the disease: the Schilling test. In this test, the patient is given an oral dose of radioactive vitamin B12, followed by an injection of regular vitamin B12. If intrinsic factor is present, any radioactive vitamin B12 absorbed will show up in the urine.

This vitamin is unique among the B vitamins in that its main sources are animal foods. For this reason, vegetarians are more likely to be B12 deficient. Birth control pills also cause a loss of this vitamin, a particularly bad situation. When a woman goes off the pill and becomes pregnant, she then starts her pregnancy with a vitamin B12 deficiency. Even with usual pre-natal supplementation it has been shown that the mother's stores of vitamin B12 drop dramatically during pregnancy. Imagine her status when she goes into pregnancy deficient and takes only the usual amounts of supplementation.

Injectable B12 comes in two forms, the more common cyanocobalamine, and the less commonly used hydroxy-cobalamine. The cyanocobalamine is excreted from the body fairly rapidly, so that a single 1000 microgram injection will last only about a month. The same amount of hydroxycobalamine will remain in the body for about a year. If your physician decides to use vitamin B12 injections, you should request the hydroxy-cobalamine form. A once-a-year injection of this form of the vitamin is probably cheaper than the Schilling test.

Shingles, medically termed Zoster, is a severe viral illness caused by the same virus that causes chickenpox. It frequently results in painful lesions that remain painful for years. Studies in India have shown that large doses of vitamin B12, given frequently (daily) will abort the pain and complications of this disease. I have found that shingles responds predictably and quickly to nutritional therapy, but only if treatment is begun within three days of onset of pain, about the time the first blisters appear.

Alcohol and tobacco team up to produce a frequent cause of blindness, alcohol tobacco amblyopia. I have seen this disease fairly often. Caught in time, it will respond to treatment with hydroxycobalamine. The cyano-form is not effective. This disease is a classic example of a disease reaching a point of no return. A nutritionally-caused disease may not respond to nutritional therapy if it is applied too late. Neither does surgery work once the patient is dead.

In any case, be aware that whenever mental or nerve disease exists, whenever growth or healing is slow, whenever pregnancy occurs, and whenever birth control pills or excessive alcohol are consumed, vitamin B12 deficiency is a possibility. Of course, with alcohol, the source is important since yeast generously produces all of the complex of B vitamins. Wine and beer would probably not cause a deficiency unless they were used to excess, thus producing a fatty liver. Distilled spirits, however, do not have these redeeming qualities. How many cases of senility are due to this deficiency? We will never know unless tests are performed. As with all diagnoses, awareness makes the diagnosis more likely.

Folic Acid

RECOMMENDED DAILY ALLOWANCES:

Infants	0.1 mg
Children	0.2 mg
Adults	0.4 mg
Pregnant	0.8 mg

MAJOR DIETARY SOURCES:
Liver
Wheat bran
Asparagus
Beet greens
Kale
Endive
Spinach
Turnips
MAJOR FUNCTIONS:
Red blood cell formation
RNA and DNA synthesis

Folic acid was first discovered in the leaves (foliage) of spinach, hence its name. It is one of two antianemic vitamins stored in the liver.

Folic acid deficiencies are common. Studies two decades ago

confirmed that folic acid deficiencies existed in 75 percent of women who had spontaneous abortions. It was these studies that caused the addition of folic acid to prenatal vitamins. Other studies have shown that pregnant women not treated with supplemental folic acid show deficiencies in as many as 94 percent of those tested. Sixteen percent show severe deficiencies. When you look at the number of birth-related problems associated with folic acid deficiency, you can see the reason for concern: toxemia, abruptio placentae, premature birth, and post-partum hemorrhage.

Like B12, folic acid requirements are increased with the use of birth control pills. Again, this sets the potential mother up for real problems when she does decide to become pregnant, since she enters a period of great need for the vitamin with reduced stores. Unfortunately, the FDA restricts the amount of folic acid available without prescription to 0.4 milligrams, which is only half the RDA for pregnant women. The FDA has chosen to protect the public against a rare disease, leaving a common deficiency uncorrected, to the great risk to millions of unborn children. The FDA decision is foolish, since women with pernicious anemia do not get pregnant! Pregnant women, and those taking the pill, should get a prescription from their physician and take several milligrams of folic acid daily. The risk of masking B12 deficiency in pregnancy is minimal.

Folic acid deficiency can develop very rapidly after severe trauma, burns, or surgery, when considerable cell division is occurring. Since vitamin C is necessary for folic acid to be converted to its active form, and since vitamin C demands are also greatly increased during trauma, there is a double danger of deficiency after injury. Vitamin B12 is also necessary for folic acid to be converted to its active form.

This complex interaction between the various vitamins is just another reason why isolated vitamin therapy may be unwise. It is also a good reason why the FDA's restriction of folic acid in vitamin supplements is unwise, preventing a rare complication while ignoring a common deficiency with widespread implications.

Unfortunately, folic acid can cure the anemia due to vitamin B12 deficiency, and leave the progressive nerve damage unchecked. Apparently, it takes at least 1 milligram of folic acid to mask pernicious anemia, whereas 0.4 milligrams is usually sufficient to treat a deficiency. For this reason, federal law forbids the sale of folic acid without prescription except in small amounts. However, you should notice that the amount restricted by law does not even meet the RDA set by the USDA. It would be nice if tablets of perhaps 5 milligrams were available, at least by prescription.

Like other B vitamins, folic acid has been demonstrated to cure some schizophrenic patients. Their interaction is so complex, however, that no clear pattern emerges. It is sufficient to be aware that mental illness can be due to vitamin deficiencies.

Although folic acid is plentiful in the foods listed above, it is quite easily destroyed by heat, air, and light. It is also water soluble, so that cooked greens will have lost most of their vitamin value unless the water is also consumed. The "pot liquor" left after the greens are eaten is perhaps more nutritious than the greens themselves. Don't pour it out: drink it down. We have found that many of the greens traditionally cooked are delicious raw in a salad. This is especially true of spinach, one of the richest sources of folic acid. Also, fresh greens would obviously be more nutritious than canned. Freshly frozen greens would be a good second choice. Canned greens may not be worth the effort from a nutritional point of view, since careful studies have shown that canned vegetables have lost about 60 percent of their nutritional value. The loss for frozen vegetables is under 20 percent, depending on how long they have been frozen.

Some patients with visual problems have been shown to improve rapidly with folic acid. Certainly, a therapeutic trial of folic acid in patients with unexplained visual loss is justified. I do not mean the indiscriminate use of vitamins to avoid a good medical and neurological workup: I am referring to the patient with a normal appearing eye who has no obvious cause for his poor vision. Vitamin therapy may be a more logical and less expensive approach. More importantly, the statistics of deficiencies are on the side to nutritional therapy.

Take children: folic acid is necessary for growth and development, yet how many children do you know who enjoy those foods rich in folic acid? Look at that list again. From the average child's point of view, a less appetizing list could not be devised! A study at one school found that 99 percent of the children had diets deficient in folic acid. Look again: folic acid deficiency is very close to home.

Fortunately, folic acid is synthesized in the gut by friendly bacteria. If supplied with PABA (para-aminobenzoic acid), it is very readily synthesized, a good reason for adding PABA to your nutritional supplementation, and a simple way to bypass the FDA restrictions.

Pantothenic Acid

RECOMMENDED DAILY ALLOWANCES:

Infants	3 mg.
Children	5 mg.
Adults	10 mg.
Pregnant	10 mg.

MAJOR SOURCES:
  Liver
  Kidney
  Heart
  Brewer's yeast
  Sunflower seeds
  Peanuts
  Buckwheat flour

MAJOR FUNCTIONS:
  Adrenal gland function
  Antibody production
  Muscle function
  Anti-stress function
  Bowel function
  Protects against radiation

This vitamin was named because it is almost everywhere, and a deficiency is virtually impossible. Or was impossible before modern food production and storage. Pantothenic acid is a classic example of how our modern diet no longer supplies what we think it supplies.

Methyl bromide is a fumigant used by virtually all food processors and storage facilities because it will kill virtually anything, and disappears without a trace once the storage area is ventilated. Methyl bromide is also used to sterilize soil before planting seed, because it will destroy wild seed in the soil, as well as rodents and other pests. What could be better? No roaches, no mice, just good clean food? Unfortunately, methyl bromide also destroys every trace of pantothenic acid that may have been in the food. So throw away your tables of nutritional values: if you are eating commercially stored foods, you are getting virtually no pantothenic acid in your diet.

This startling discovery was made in Japan where patients were developing symptoms of nerve and optic degeneration, expressed by loss of vision, spinal cord lesions, irritability, and constipation. By coincidence, a man exposed to methyl bromide developed similar symptoms, and further investigations proved that their symptoms could be cured by injections of pantothenic acid. The connection between methyl bromide fumigation of food storage areas and diseases consistent with pantothenic acid deficiency has not been proven. What has been proven is that methyl bromide destroys this vitamin, and that this vitamin is essential for nerve and muscle function, and resistance to infection and stress.

Humans deprived of pantothenic acid develop deficiency symptoms within two weeks. This clearly shows how important this vitamin is, and how little of it we are able to store. Deficiency symptoms include the following, many common to other B vitamins: loss of appetite, constipation, irritability, quarrelsomeness, fatigue, frequent respiratory infections, and finally a burning sensation of the feet. Without pantothenic acid, we cannot withstand stress, nor can we make antibodies. Coenzyme A, necessary for production of energy in the body, is made from this vitamin. Without it, muscle action will cease.

Studies in Europe have demonstrated a strong relationship between low blood levels of pantothenic acid and arthritis, including remission of arthritis with treatment with the vitamin, and recurrence when the vitamin was no longer added to the diet.

German research has shown that the addition of pantothenic acid to treatment with certain antibiotics toxic to the kidneys and hearing will reduce the toxic side effects. Patients undergoing general surgery suffer several days with abdominal gas pains until the intestines again function properly. The addition of this vitamin has been shown to restore bowel function quickly. For example, the hospital stay of those taking no supplemental pantothenic acid was fourteen days, while those taking the vitamin had an average stay of only two days. Since hospital costs are about $250 per day, the administration of about twenty cents worth of pantothenic acid saved $2500 in hospital costs. Good nutrition does not cost, it pays.

Incidentally, although the recommended allowance of pantothenic acid is 10 milligrams per day, 250 milligrams was used in this study. Many scientists have concluded that certain vitamins were ineffective when the dose used in their study was clearly insufficient. For example, how can a study purporting that 250 milligrams of vitamin C is ineffective against viral infections be meaningful when it has been clearly proven that during such illnesses it takes several grams of the vitamin daily to maintain usual blood levels? All vitamins were at one time produced by our ancestors. For them, they were not vitamins, they were enzymes.

And their bodies produced more when more was needed. We are like a diabetic who must adjust his own dosage of insulin in regard to vitamins: we have to adjust our dose to the need. For certain vitamins, foods simply cannot provide the quantity needed for optimum health.

One must be constantly amazed when one sees evidence of diverse effects of various vitamins. For example, who would have thought that giving pantothenic acid and calcium would stop bruxism, the grinding of teeth in sleep. Many people are plagued with this affliction, thought to be related to nervousness and pent-up emotions. Well it might, but the fact still remains that dietary supplements have been able to end the practice. Since both calcium and pantothenic acid affect nerve function, it could also be that their nervousness was due to malnutrition.

Unfortunately, pantothenic acid does not have the glamour associated with other vitamins. The fact that it is found in high concentration in active tissues (muscle) and many foods (unprocessed, of course) is evidence that it is needed. Were we to all raise our own food, and store it carefully, deficiency would be unlikely. But in a world that uses methyl bromide to protect food in storage from vermin, do not expect to get your pantothenic acid from your diet. It isn't there.

Biotin

RECOMMENDED DAILY ALLOWANCE:

Infants	0.05 mg.
Children	0.15 mg.
Adults	0.30 mg.
Pregnant	0.30 mg.

MAJOR SOURCES:
  Yeast
  Liver
  Egg yoke
  Whole grain cereals
  Nuts
  Fish
MAJOR FUNCTIONS:
  Involved in health of all cells
  Carbohydrate, protein and fat metabolism
  Necessary for growth
  Skin health
  Biotin is an unusual vitamin in that it is synthesized in the

intestines of both man and animals. A complete deficiency is therefore rare, and perhaps almost impossible. Almost.

Since bacteria in a healthy gut produce this vitamin, antibiotics which kill these helpful bacteria stop production of biotin. Prolonged antibiotic usage has resulted in deficiency conditions. Synthetic diets such as used for severely ill patients or for weight control will quickly induce biotin deficiency unless biotin is included in the formula.

Raw eggs contain a protein that combines with biotin so that it cannot be digested. Deficiency states have been produced by persons on a raw egg diet. Cooked eggs do not destroy biotin. Persons deficient in biotin generally have skin disease, especially seborrheic dermatitis (dandruff). The advent of synthetic diets for hospitalized patients who cannot eat has resulted in several cases of biotin deficiency. There has been at least one case of severe suicidal depression which quickly responded to biotin supplements. Infants with seborrheic dermatitis may respond to biotin injections, or to liver added to the diet of their nursing mother. Renal dialysis patients become biotin deficient and develop suicidal tendencies.

Biotin has been proven by the New York Academy of Sciences (1986) to significantly reduce blood sugar levels in diabetics. My personal experience is that 1000 mcg of biotin daily does in fact lower blood sugar levels in some diabetics. The same dosage of biotin is effective in a substantial percentage of patients with glaucoma in significantly reducing intraocular pressures. The effect seems to occur fairly rapidly, within one or two days, and thereby justifies a therapeutic trial of biotin.

Unfortunately, those foods richest in biotin are not common in our diet, either because of preference, or expense. Supplementation has been beneficial to some. Since everyone varies in their need for each vitamin, the best course would be to supplement your diet with biotin in its isolated form, and see if you notice any benefits over a period of time. If you notice improvement, either change your diet to include those foods rich in biotin, or use a biotin supplement.

Inositol

RDA NOT ESTABLISHED
MAJOR SOURCES:
    Beef heart
    Beef brain
    Bulgar wheat

Brown rice
Brewer's yeast
Molasses
Soybeans and soy lecithin
MAJOR FUNCTIONS:
Unknown: Found in high concentration in brain, stomach, kidney, liver, and spleen
Acts with vitamin E to repair nerve damage in muscular dystrophy.
Acts to lower blood cholesterol.
Acts to break up fat deposits.

Inositol was proven to be a vitamin in 1956. Whether supplements are needed has not been proven conclusively.

Inositol occurs in extremely high concentrations in the human brain. It is synthesized by bacteria in the intestine, and perhaps by human tissue cells also. Because of this, necessity for inclusion in the diet has not been proven to the satisfaction of the FDA.

That doesn't mean that the addition of inositol to the diet has no effect, for it most certainly has, and the effects are beneficial: Inositol in doses of up to 3 grams daily has been shown in several studies to reduce blood cholesterol in those patients with elevated cholesterol. It may be particularly effective in diabetics. For those interested in trying this approach, be aware that the initial result may be an elevation of blood cholesterol as deposits are flushed out. As cholesterol deposits are dissolved, they must be transported to the liver by the blood, so a test for blood cholesterol levels will indicate an elevation. Occasionally, a patient with elevated cholesterol levels will develop cholesterol deposits in the eyelids, which appear as yellow plaques. I have one patient with these whom I have been treating nutritionally. Although her blood cholesterol levels have not decreased, the size of the plaques has shrunk approximately 75 percent over the past year. Inositol's ability to break up abnormal fat deposits has also been demonstrated in liver cirrhosis. This effect is more pronounced when combined with choline, another related vitamin B factor. Inositol also acts in harmony with vitamin E and biotin. Inositol's effect in lowering cholesterol is almost parallel to that of vitamin C, but so far it has not been proven that the two act together in producing that effect.

Inositol also tends to inhibit tumor growth. In this regard, it acts like other antioxidant vitamins.

One of the problems in study of this vitamin is its complex inter-relation with other factors, most now unknown. Currently, one thing is certain: inositol works in conjunction with other vitamins.

Therefore, it should not be taken alone, but especially, along with vitamin C, vitamin E, biotin, and choline. Incidentally, granular lecithin is the most effective and inexpensive form of lecithin. Unfortunately, it is also the most inconvenient to take, and along with all forms of processed lecithin is highly oxidized. Possibly the best source of lecithin is whole soybeans, which can be grown as a garden vegetable, and are cooked and eaten like lima beans. The pods should be picked when full, but while the beans are still green, and cooked in boiling water a few minutes so that the pods can be opened. The taste lies between a green lima bean and boiled peanuts.

Choline

RDA NOT ESTABLISHED
MAJOR SOURCES:
>   Beef liver
>   Brewer's yeast
>   Fish
>   Peanuts
>   Soybeans
>   Lecithin
>   Egg yolks

MAJOR FUNCTIONS:
>   Production of acetylcholine (which transmits nerve impulses)
>   Liver function

Choline is a major component of lecithin, in which it is bound to phosphate compounds. The other major component of lecithin is inositol. Although an official MDR has not been established, that does not mean that it is not essential. It is. Choline if the major component of acetylcholine, the neuromuscular messenger. Pantothenic acid (another B vitamin) is needed for synthesis of acetylcholine. Thus, without choline and pahtothenic acid, nerves cannot transmit their messages.

Choline enables the liver to handle fat droplets in the blood, such as occurs after a fatty meal or during fasting or weight loss. Without choline in even a single meal, fatty deposits in the liver will occur. A fatty liver is not able to efficiently perform its other vital functions. Fatty liver is also a common problem in those who excessively drink alcohol.

Choline has other beneficial effects: given to hypertensive patients, it reduces the pressure within three weeks, especially in those with symtomatic hypertension. Choline acts with folic acid, vitamin B12, and methionine to build immunity to infection. Choline deficiency during pregnancy results in lifelong susceptibility to infection and cancer in laboratory animals. It may do the same in humans.

Choline is plentiful in human milk. It is absent in cow's milk. An infant fed a cow's milk formula will be choline deficient, and perhaps made susceptible to infections for the rest of his life. This is another strong point in favor of breast feeding. Choline is also plentiful in soybean protein and in lecithin, so soybean milk would be better than cow's milk as a substitute for human milk in nursing infants.

In fact, an ideal drink for children is the soybean protein supplement which has been enriched with methionine. Lecithin is used as the emulsifier in these nutritional beverages. Since soybean protein is deficient in methionine, it is important that the product you select has added methionine. Since choline deficiency affects offspring, soybean products which are rich in choline would be a wise choice for expectant mothers. Lecithin capsules or granules are also an excellent source of choline. Since lecithin is an excellent emulsifier, making fats soluble in water; it is commonly used in many prepared foods. This is one example of an additive being beneficial to our health. The other side of processed lecithin is that it is also oxidized. The best sources of lecithin are unprocessed foods.

PABA

RDA NOT ESTABLISHED
MAJOR SOURCES:
 Beef liver
 Brewer's yeast
 Eggs
 Yogurt
 Whole grains
 Molasses
MAJOR FUNCTIONS:
 Protein metabolism
 Enables intestinal bacterial to produce folic acid
 Involved in blood formation
 Absorbs ultraviolet radiation (prevents sunburn)
 May prevent skin cancer
 Necessary for use of pantothenic acid
 PABA is short for para-aminobenzoic acid. It is part of the

vitamin, folic acid, but also acts alone as a co-enzyme. Intestinal bacteria can use PABA to synthesize folic acid.

PABA combines in the intestine with the same proteins as sulfa drugs. Thus, prolonged use of sulfa drugs may produce PABA deficiency, and along with it a folic and pantothenic acid deficiency. It is interesting that the toxic side effects of sulfa drugs, and some diuretics similar to sulfa drugs, are the same as the symptoms of deficiencies of these vitamins. Unfortunately, PABA administration makes sulfa drugs ineffective. If your physician gives you a sulfa drug in treatment of an infection (most commonly a urinary tract infection), you must stop taking the PABA if you want the medicine to be effective.

PABA prevents skin changes due to aging, possibly a result of its absorption of harmful ultraviolet light. That capability may make it useful in preventing skin cancer, which is known to be more common in areas of intense solar radiation. PABA is the effective ingredients in many suntan lotions designed to screen ultraviolet light. In combination with pantothenic acid, choline, and folic acid, PABA has been used successfully in treatment of gray hair. I cannot personally vouch for this effect. PABA has estrogen-like effects and may be useful in controlling menopausal symptoms.

Deficiency of PABA may result in extreme fatigue, nausea, eczema, anemia, gray hair, infertility, vitiligo, and/or loss of libido.

Tablets with more than 30 milligrams of PABA require a prescription. One hundred milligrams daily is safe, but very large doses are potentially harmful to the heart, kidneys, and liver. PABA has recently become popular in the (probably mistaken) belief that it will prevent sunburn if taken orally. There is no proof of this. It is extremely effective when applied to the skin as a 5 percent solution in ethyl alcohol, and this may well be absorbed through the skin. For those interested in preventing sunburn, I would recommend use of vitamin E, beta carotene, vitamin C and aspirin, instead. As with the other vitamins, PABA is most effective in a balanced formula.

XIX.
The Essential
Mineral Elements

Our bodies are made from the earth, and most of the minerals found in the soil are necessary for life. Aside from the fact that the Bible proclaims that we were made from clay, it should be obvious to anyone that every atom within our bodies comes from what we eat, plus what we breathe and absorb through the skin. Ions of metallic elements function as catalysts due to their electron charge plus the physical size of the metal ion in solution, and thus influence chemical reactions within the body to their proper direction. These elements serve as structural elements (bone), parts of enzymes (vitamin B12), co-factors for metabolic processes (zinc, selenium, chromium, etc.), and for mundane things like maintaining blood volume (sodium).

For the purposes of this book, I have divided the elements into three groups. First, the structural elements: calcium, phosphorus, magnesium, potassium, sodium, chlorine, and sulfur. These are all required in relatively large quantities, up to several grams per day. Second, the lesser elements: iron, manganese, copper, zinc, and silicon. These are extremely important, but mere milligrams are required per day. Third, the trace elements: iodine, selenium, chromium, fluorine, molybdenum, cobalt, and lithium. The trace elements are required in microgram quantities. There is a fourth group of trace elements that are present in the human body, but their function is unknown: boron, lead, strontium, nickel, bromine, germanium, and vanadium to name a few.

The structural elements are plentiful in fresh vegetables and milk. The lesser and trace elements are frequently missing from the soil and food due to poor farming techniques over the past century. What we have not lost from erosion, we have lost by replacing only nitrates, potassium, calcium, phosphorus, and magnesium with commercial fertilizers. The other elements that were present in the soil have long since been taken up by the plants, and then removed by harvest. Had we used organic farming methods, mulching with organic garbage, leaves and organic residues, we would have been replacing those lost elements as we improved fertility. Organic mulching works because, although most organic materials are not rich in the required minerals, they do contain trace amounts of these minerals, and in time the levels will build up.

We need to recognize that the topsoil is (was) a living organism; it is not a vehicle to hold the roots of plants so that they will stand upright under the sun. Through the use of chemical fertilizers, we have denied earthworms a decent meal and then added injury to insult by the use of pesticides. Earthworms are not just something we fish with: they cultivate the soil, release minerals to the topsoil, and loosen the soil for rapid penetration of rain and air. The rich topsoil present when our forefathers came to America was several feet deep, but has dwindled to a mere few inches, and is no longer the black loam we once had. Obviously, nature has a way of building soil. We need to learn to work with nature. There is no way to win when we struggle against her. As an aside, I wonder how much of the flooding of the midwest these past two years is a result of the loss of our topsoil which would have acted as a sponge to hold the water where it fell. When the soil is healthy, it catches the spring rains and holds the water so that there is a slow steady release throughout the dry summer.

Unless you practice organic gardening, and additionally augment your mulch with nutrient-rich products such as kelp or green sand, you cannot expect your garden to fully supply the trace elements you need. Nevertheless, your home garden will produce food far superior to what you will find in your grocery store. This is true in part because much produce must be picked green in order for it to be shipped without damage, and then is forced to ripen by the use of gas or chemicals. The red tomato you buy at your grocery store is not ripe, it is merely a red tomato. If you have ever eaten a vine ripened tomato you know the difference.

Mineral deficiencies are very common. The Senate Select Committee on Nutrition concluded that 99 percent of the American population is deficient in at least some elements. The chances are great that you, too, lack some important elements, either structural, lesser, or trace. Studies in Atlanta and Boston have concluded that about 85 percent of the population is zinc deficient. Persons who have heart attacks are almost all deficient in selenium, and usually also chromium. Hypoglycemia is epidemic today in the U.S., the inevitable result of an excess of highly refined carbohydrates (sugar and white flour) and a deficiency of chromium. As you would expect, excellent sources of chromium are bran and unrefined sugar, provided by God with the food just where it was needed, and removed by the food processors so that the food would store well. Even the vermin know better than to eat that stuff.

However, it should be added at this point that the symptoms of hypoglycemia can be duplicated by Candida albicans overgrowth in the gut, or by food allergy. Food allergy is made worse by Candida infestation, and the overgrowth of candida is in turn made worse by diets rich in processed foods, and by antibiotic useage.

Additionally, although raw sugar is a rich source of chromium, brown sugar is not. Brown sugar is a processed product made with white sugar and molasses.

Finally, since iron and chromium both bind to the same blood protein (ferritin), an excess of iron leads to a chromium deficiency, and thus may be a major cause of adult onset diabetes. Furthermore, a chromium deficiency will result in higher blood sugar levels, and will cause a further loss of body chromium.

Replacing trace elements is not too difficult, however. Switching from mined salt to sea salt will supply some of your needs. Ocean salt is rich in the trace elements that have been eroded into the sea. Use the sea salt just as you would regular salt, anytime you would ordinarily use salt. Since what passes for sea salt at many health food stores is evaporated salt which has had its trace elements removed for sale separately, you will have to find a supplier and have an analysis run. If it is rich in magnesium and has little iron or aluminum it is genuine.

A second method of obtaining trace elements is to include sea foods, such as seaweed and kelp, in your regular diet. All seafoods are rich in the trace elements naturally present in the sea, and contain the beneficial elements in higher concentrations than does sea salt. Living organisms concentrate elements found in the environment, with each step in the food chain further concentrating the minerals.

Unfortunately, toxic wastes are also concentrated in the food chain. Of course, not only sea life has been affected by our pollution: until DDT was banned, our eagle population was disappearing because the DDT was preventing the eagles from laying eggs with hard shells. Since we are at the end of the food chain, we will be the final recipient of our pollution. Our sins will return to us many times magnified. This is not the result of a vengeful God, this is nothing more than the working out of natural laws which parallel spiritual laws. The physical realm is merely a reflection of the spiritual world, and all spiritual laws have parallel physical laws. That, however, is the topic of another book.

A third source for minerals is alfalfa, which sends its roots over forty feet deep, picking up trace minerals still present at depth. Most plants have shallow root systems, so will not pick up these elements. Of course, where the alfalfa grows will make a major difference. Alfalfa is an excellent source of minerals, plus it is an excellent source of fiber. I would recommend taking about six tablets daily, especially on those days in which seafoods are not eaten. Incidentally, alfalfa leaves will stimulate a garden to grow much better, possibly due to trace elements in the leaves. Needless to say, don't buy alfalfa tablets to put in your garden! Buy alfalfa hay, instead. Not only does alfalfa make your garden grow, but researchers at Shaklee Corporation have found that alfalfa leaves contain something, not yet identified, which stimulates growth in young animals. I believe alfalfa should especially be included in the diet of children as well as adults. Many arthritics have found relief through the use of alfalfa, plus other supplements. A cheaper, and tastier, source of the nutrients in alfalfa is alfalfa sprouts which you can buy in your grocery store, or can sprout at home. They do well added to salads, or added to hamburger meat and cooked.

A fourth rich source of minor and trace minerals is Spirulina, a type of algae that grows in the mineral lakes of Mexico. This algae is an excellent source for complete protein plus minerals. Its main disadvantages are its cost, and its taste. It smells and tastes like what it is: scum from stagnant water. Nutritious it is, and it will support life with it as the only source of food. In fact, one Japanese researcher has eaten nothing but Spirulina for over a decade, and remains very healthy and vigorous. His dedication is beyond repute! The tablet form is fairly easy to take, but you have to acquire a taste for the powder form! That, I can assure you, is more easily said than done.

The lesser and trace elements are more easily absorbed and used by the body if they are bound to organic molecules before ingestion. Minerals obtained from natural sources such as Spirulina, seafood, alfalfa, and yeast will be easily assimilated. Inorganic minerals are cheaper, and many mineral tablets use this form. Unfortunately, you cannot use them effectively.

All of the lesser end trace elements are essential to life in small quantities, but are toxic in excess. It is easily possible to take toxic doses of these elements. Some, like calcium, will not easily be absorbed to excess. Others, like iron, will be absorbed to excess only if the natural diet is supplemented with iron, as it is in America. If you get most of your elements from natural food sources you will be very unlikely to get an excess.

A balance is necessary. Calcium, phosphorous, and magnesium make up the mineral crystals of bone. Dolomite tablets do not contain phosphorus, do usually contain cadmium (a heavy metal poison), and are poorly absorbed. However, if you eat a fair portion of processed foods you will be getting ample phosphorus, since it is added freely to control acidity. Bone meal, although balanced, may contain radioactive strontium from nuclear bomb testing during the 1950s, plus it usually contains toxic levels of lead. This is a diminishing problem, but certainly one you should be aware of. Incidentally, extra dietary calcium will help rid the bones of radioactive strontium. I think it is ill advised to take calcium without taking magnesium.

The approach I would recommend to assure you are getting enough of the essential elements is to switch to sea salt (genuine, of course) for all your salt needs. Of course, if you are on a salt-free diet sea salt cannot be used. But some salt will be used, and that should be sea salt. Next, include seafoods at least weekly in your diet. Freshwater fish do not count. Using seaweed and kelp as flavorings should be considered. The taste may take some getting used to, but the Japanese do so daily. Six or more alfalfa tablets will not only provide trace elements, but fiber as well. Alfalfa sprouts are preferable to tablets. You probably should take a mineral supplement tablet which uses organically-bound minerals. The tablets should provide at least the following minerals: zinc, 20 milligrams; chromium, 200 micrograms; selenium, 200 micrograms; iodine, 100 micrograms; vanadium, 500 micrograms; and manganese, 20 milligrams. Ideally, your supplements should also include about 50 micrograms each of cobalt, molybdenum, and lithium. Organically-bound silicon is an essential mineral, but the amount needed is unknown. Probably over a gram is needed daily. Alfalfa is the richest readily available source of silicon. "Willard water" is another source of silicon. All natural food fiber is rich in silicon. However, note that high fiber bread made with cellulose (wood pulp) is not a source of any of the trace elements found in natural fiber. Iron and copper should not be taken unless there is a documented deficiency.

No general mineral tablet is going to contain sufficient amounts of potassium, calcium, phosphorus, or magnesium; to do so would make the tablet too large to swallow. Potassium and magnesium are plentiful in green, leafy vegetables. Calcium and phosphorus are abundant in dairy products. The best potassium supplements are available only by prescription, but all whole foods are rich in potassium. Potassium deficiency is more a problem of sodium excess, and magnesium deficiency, than of actual potassium deficiency. Because processed food is rich in phosphorus there is usually no need to take supplemental phosphorus. In fact, it is ill advised.

The best product currently on the market is made by Advanced Medical Nutrition, Inc. They sell only to physicians, or to persons authorized by physicians. Basic Preventive™ is available complete, without iron, without copper, or without copper or iron. The company has an 800 number. It is also available from Bio-Zoe, Inc., P.O. Box 49, Waynesville, NC 28786-0049.

If a hair analysis (available from Bio-Zoe, Inc., above) indicates a generalized mineral deficiency, there are several products which will supply minerals. Two of the best are Spirulina, and Body Toddy™. Body Toddy™ is a high mineral water which is manufactured from lignite, a prehistoric vegetable deposit between peat and brown coal in consistency. In the manufacture of Body Toddy™ lignite is ground up and soaked in catalysed water (water which has been altered by injecting electrons into it to lower its surface tension) and allowing it to soak for an extended period of time. The material is then filtered leaving the dissolved minerals in the water. There are other similar products on the market, but only Body Toddy™ uses catalysed water. It is an excellent source of selenium, containing about 27 mcg per ounce, and is one of the few sources that contains almost all of the essential minerals in a fairly balanced product. Its main weakness is a relative lack of zinc, chromium, and manganese. That is, relative to the other minerals. I therefore recommend additional supplementation of these minerals, if a deficiency exists, when using the Body Toddy.™ In my own practice, I do not use this product without first doing a hair analysis, and I follow my patients with hair analyses every few months while they are taking it. The usual dose is ½ to 3 ounces per day, taken with citrus juice or V-8™ juice. It is only fair to warn the reader the Body Toddy™ is very concentrated, and tastes terrible. Nevertheless, the results I am getting in correcting mineral deficiency diseases is somewhat spectacular. Body Toddy™ has a high zeta potential; and, being colloidal, is very well absorbed. Body Toddy™ may be ordered from Bio-Zoe, Inc., P.O. Box 49, Waynesville, North Carolina 28786.

XX.
The Structural Elements

Calcium is important both as a structural element and for nerve and muscle function. Mention calcium, and immediately strong bones and teeth come to mind. And well it should, because calcium composes 10 percent of the weight of bone, and 25 percent of the weight of teeth. But the calcium in bone and teeth is not like rock in a stone wall for it is constantly being exchanged with calcium in the blood. Bone is not solid as you might suppose, it is made up of thin sheets of mineral placed so that there is maximum strength with minimum weight. As you change the stresses put on your bones, they will slowly change shape over a period of weeks to meet the new demands. Strength is more than muscle, it is also in the architecture of bone. So throw away any idea of a static skeleton, it is a very dynamic and living structure.

Calcium is absolutely essential in many body functions, including all nerve and muscle actions, clotting of blood, and many enzyme actions. The body has many mechanisms for maintaining blood calcium levels within very narrow limits. Additionally, it will automatically adjust absorption from food so that you cannot easily get too much by supplementation.

Currently, the accepted RDA for calcium is 800 milligrams for adults, increased to 1500 milligrams for children and pregnant or nursing women. However, recent research suggests that the amount to maintain positive calcium balance should be about twice this lower figure, especially for women over 40. This is most likely due to a pathological dependency state (the result of our distorted diet), since people eating a primitive diet exhibit positive calcium balance (meaning that their diet contains excess calcium) with only 300 milligrams of calcium a day. In spite of this, I still recommend supplementation with at least 300 milligrams of calcium daily. Supplementation with 3 grams of calcium daily can lead to toxic side effects.

The average American diet includes only about 600 milligrams of calcium. Many ingest much less than that. As a result, calcium levels in the blood necessary for muscle and nerve function. This is caused by increased parathyroid hormone secretion, and results in higher levels of ionized calcium in the blood. This, in turn, may result in hypertension and abnormal calcium deposits both in arterial walls and as kidney stones. Drugs called calcium channel blockers are used to treat the hypertension caused by the excess calcium ion levels, but the same goal can be accomplished by ingesting more calcium to correct the diet deficiency. A better solution is to modify the diet to exclude processed fats, and to supplement the diet with essential fatty acids (evening primrose oil being an excellent source). This change will allow the body to repair defective cell membranes so that they are no longer defective (permeable or leaky). Healthy cell membranes do not need calcium channel blockers to keep excess calcium and sodium from entering the cells.

Fortunately, bone is a large reservoir for calcium. Unfortunately, the weakened bones are easily broken. The common event of elderly citizens falling and breaking a hip is the end result of chronic calcium deficiency. In fact, many orthopedic surgeons have concluded that it is the bone breaking that causes the fall, not the other way around.

Calcium is found in abundance in milk and cheese. It is also abundant in dark leafy vegetables. In recent years phosphate-rich carbonated drinks have replaced milk as a beverage, which not only reduces the amount of calcium taken into the body, but actually depletes the body of calcium. Milk consumption has also been reduced by those who consider it too high in calories.

I had myself considered milk as less than perfect, and consumed less than a glass a month. I did eat cheese at least once or twice a week, but not in quantity. A few months ago I listened to a physician lecturer, who claimed that it was impossible to design a diet that met the RDA of all recognized nutrients. I doubted that, but an analysis of my own diet revealed that I was getting only 50 percent of the RDA of calcium. It also revealed that I was getting only about 50 percent of the vitamin C, and 10 percent of the vitamin E. I can assure you that my diet was far superior to that of most Americans, and still it was woefully deficient.

This jolted my thinking, and I began looking around for a palatable source of calcium. In the process, I discovered an instant protein product made from soybeans, which was also a rich source of calcium. Mixed with milk, it supplied 80 percent of my RDA. Add two calcium/magnesium tablets, and you have your 100 percent. Actually, that one serving, plus my 50 percent, would put me over the 100 percent level. But since I had had a deficiency for decades, it was prudent to increase my intake to well over the RDA. There were other reasons for selecting the instant protein, major among which was the fact that soybean protein has been proven to reduce blood cholesterol, and mine was much higher than desirable. Also, I selected a product which has methionine added to the soybean protein, making it a complete and balanced protein.

The improvement in our family's health was almost immediate. The real payoff for me came about two months later: my blood pressure, which had been impossible to control medically, moved well into the normal range. About two days after I discovered this happy fact, there was an article in the *Journal of the American Medical Association* demonstrating that calcium supplementation at 1 gram per day results in a lowered blood pressure. Other studies have shown that 2 grams of calcium daily will reduce blood cholesterol. It is studies such as these that suggest that we either are consuming too little calcium, or have habits that are depleting our bodies of usable calcium. Please note, however, that 3 grams of calcium daily is toxic.

Calcium deficiency most obviously results in osteoporosis and osteomalacia. This may appear as spontaneous collapse of vertebrae, and as chronic back pain. Joint and bone pain also are associated with chronic calcium deficiency. Muscle cramps usually mean calcium deficiency, but may also be the result of vitamin E or magnesium deficiency. Nervousness, insomnia, depression, and heart palpitations round out the picture.

Interestingly, if a person has multiple deficiencies, calcium supplementation may divert that small amount of vitamin C available to bone growth, and result in symptoms of vitamin C deficiency. I have seen this in one patient. This is just one more argument in favor of a broad-based nutritional program.

Phosphorus is a mineral companion with calcium in bone. Additionally, it is part of one of the systems that buffers body acids to maintain pH. Phosphorus is the major constituent in high energy molecules that we use for actual muscle and nerve function. Lecithin is a rich source of phosphorus.

Phosphorus deficiencies result in weak bones, poor growth, and reduced nerve function. Deficiencies are rare, because phosphates are added to so many processed foods to control acidity. In fact, most people probably get far too much of this element. Excess phosphorus will reduce calcium absorption, and is probably the major reason so many people are calcium deficient today. Food sources are whole grains, seeds and nuts, dairy products, fruit, and corn.

Dietary requirements are about the same as for calcium: 800 milligrams for adults, 1400 milligrams for children and pregnant or nursing women. Phosphorus supplementation is unwise without a demonstrated deficiency.

Magnesium is a lesser element of bone, but is especially important as a catalyst for many enzyme actions. It is critical in reactions involving energy production. Magnesium is necessary for proper use of vitamin E, and is a co-factor with vitamin B6 (pyridoxine). It is well known that women with toxemia of pregnancy can be treated with magnesium. Usually forgotten is the addition of pyridoxine to make the magnesium more effective. Magnesium is also active in the mechanism whereby choline prevents accumulation of cholesterol deposits in blood vessels.

A recent issue of the *New England Journal of Medicine* pointed out that pyridoxine taken in excess can produce neurological symptoms. Interestingly, the symptoms produced are those of magnesium deficiency, which could be precipitated by taking pyridoxine without also taking its cofactor, magnesium. Nutritional therapy should be balanced.

Magnesium plus pyridoxine have been clearly shown in a controlled study to reduce kidney stone formation. The dose used was 300 milligrams of magnesium and 10 milligrams of pyridoxine. About 80 percent of stone formers stopped producing kidney stones on this simple treatment. Part of the effect is due to the competition of magnesium for oxalate. Calcium oxalate is insoluble, while magnesium oxalate freely dissolves in urine. It would seem logical for stone formers to skip the calcium, but that is not the case: calcium deficiency increases oxalate excretion. I have one patient who had for several years been passing one or two kidney stones per week. Her urologist had put her on a low calcium diet. I talked her into taking both calcium and magnesium supplements, plus other vitamin and trace elements, and she has had no stones for over two years.

The RDA for magnesium is 350 milligrams, but evidence suggests that twice that is needed. Food sources include nuts, soybeans, green vegetables, alfalfa, figs, seeds, and whole grains.

Continuous magnesium deficiency results in loss of calcium and potassium. Magnesium is necessary for the cellular pump to move vital potassium into the cell. Intracellular potassium regulates the heartbeat and nerve function. Digitalis, a drug used to treat heart failure, can be very toxic whenever a potassium deficiency exists. It has now been shown that a major cause of digitalis toxicity is magnesium deficiency, and the resultant potassium deficiency within heart muscle. A strong argument can be made for using supplemental magnesium for all cardiac patients, especially those on digitalis, since magnesium deficiency is so common. I believe that if the truth were known, many patients who are dying with cardiac failure or digitalis toxicity are dying with, and perhaps because of, a magnesium deficiency. In fact, the death rate due to cardiovascular disease is inversely proportional to the amount of magnesium in the diet. That is, the more magnesium there is in the diet, the less likely that death will occur due to cardiovascular disease. Diabetics also suffer from potassium loss, and this can be reduced with supplemental magnesium. Now that it has been proven that diabetic cataracts can be caused by vitamin E deficiency, magnesium (which works with vitamin E in its functions) should be considered as a supplement for diabetics.

Kidney stones, atherosclerosis, hypertension, heart attacks, digitalis toxicity, nervousness, depression, confusion, and premature aging are possible symptoms of magnesium deficiency. It is interesting that these symptoms are common to most of the elderly. A casual glance at the list of food sources will convince anyone that these are not common in the diet of many Americans, and especially not the elderly, who often cannot afford them.

Potassium is a major element, required in larger quantities than any other element. It is the major ion in fluids found inside the cells, while sodium is the major ion dissolved in blood. This relationship is critical for normal nerve and muscle function. When a nerve relays a message, potassium passes out of the cell, and is replaced with sodium. The atoms are restored to their former relationship before the nerve can send another message. As mentioned above, magnesium is necessary to restore the sodium/potassium balance. Potassium is plentiful in all living cells (meat or vegetable), and in fruit juices. Bananas are an excellent source, as are the peelings of potatoes. Whole grains, nuts, and milk round out the sources of potassium. Potassium salts are highly soluble in water, and end up in the water used to cook vegetables. If you use water in the cooking of vegetables, be sure to consume the water. This loss of nutrients can be reduced or prevented by cooking with a microwave oven, or by steaming vegetables. The southern way of cooking vegetables until they are mush is terrible from a nutritional point of view.

Until the mid-50s, the American diet was a high potassium,

low sodium diet. Now our diet has become high sodium, making it relatively low in potassium. The high sodium comes from processed foods, which have added sodium because we all like the taste of salt. The average American consumes eight to ten pounds of sodium a year, which comes to over 12 grams a day, and appears to be an addiction. Since our minimum sodium needs are only about 350 milligrams, most of us are consuming 3500 percent of the MDR for sodium. Talk about overdosing in minerals! The low potassium is the result of a shift away from fresh vegetables and fruit. Many physicians suspect that it is not so much our excess of sodium, as it is our relative deficiency in potassium, that is one cause of hypertension. Indeed, a century ago potassium was used effectively to reduce blood pressure and as a diuretic. It still works today. However, I believe the underlying problem is a magnesium deficiency combined with a massive overload of dietary sodium.

Potassium deficiency results in constipation, nervousness, fatigue, weakness, and low blood sugar. This sounds like the symptom list of the many patients seeking the help of their physician, perhaps even someone you know. Severe deficiencies results in sodium retention, edema, and high blood pressure. Diuretics prescribed to remove excess sodium also tend to remove potassium. Anyone taking diuretics should take potassium, plus magnesium, and shift their diet to foods rich in potassium. For me, diuretics are ineffective without supplemental potassium, and with the potassium I don't seem to need the diuretics. Supplements are unnecessary if your diet is rich in unprocessed foods.

Sodium and chlorine are both essential major minerals. Deficiencies are extremely rare, but have occurred in persons on synthetic diets. Our problem today is an excess, not a deficiency.

Sulfur is the last major element, and considered to be available in sufficient quantities in the average diet. Sulfur is similar chemically to selenium, and selenium and sulfur both are effective in topical application in controlling dandruff. This makes me suspicious that our diet does not supply enough of this essential mineral. Sulfur is necessary for healthy skin, hair, and nails. When sulfur deficiencies are present, brittle nails and hair develop. Skin rashes also occur.

Natural sources of sulfur are radishes, turnips, onions, celery, horseradish, string beans, watercress, kale, soybeans, fish and meat.

If you garden, and your soil is deficient in magnesium and sulfur, ask your agricultural agent how much Epsom salts to add to the soil to correct both deficiencies. Epsom salt is magnesium sulfate. Our soil required about one pound of Epsom salts per 1000 square feet.

XXI.
The Lesser Elements

The lesser elements are those which are needed in milligram quantities: copper, iron, manganese, silicon, vanadium, and zinc. However, silicon may soon be considered a major essential element as research continues.

Iron deficiency is considered by some to be the most common deficiency in the USA, especially among women. Men require about 10 milligrams per day, and women require 18 milligrams per day. Iron is added to many foods in an effort to reduce this perceived deficiency, but in the process males are being overdosed with iron, the result of good intentions going awry. Once hemoglobin levels are adequate, and serum ferritin is saturated, the excess iron remains unattached and ionized. This ionized iron is an extremely potent catalyst of free radicals, which we have seen is the major cause of degenerative diseases. Not only that, but chromium and iron are bound to the same blood protein, and excess iron will displace some of the chromium, which is lost through the kidneys. This loss of chromium due to ionized iron may be one cause of adult onset diabetes. After menopause, women build up their iron stores and become prey to ionized iron. In addition, widespread iron supplementation in food has caused problems for those rare individuals who absorb too much iron. The actual need for iron is much less, but the RDA assumes only 10 percent of that ingested is absorbed. Vitamin C and acid foods enhance iron absorption, and decrease dietary iron needed.

Interestingly, your body is designed to keep iron out rather than bring it in, but this defense mechanism is unable to withstand the onslaught of massive iron supplementation. Unless iron deficiency is documented by serum ferritin levels, do not try to bypass this protection by taking supplemental iron. *Do not take supplemental iron without proof of a deficiency.* If you ingest too much iron, constipation and black stools will result. You also risk significant free radical pathology.

Iron is the essential metal ion in hemoglobin, which carries oxygen in the blood. Too little iron, and you cannot make enough hemoglobin to supply oxygen to your body. The resulting anemia reduces the ability to work. Men generally have hemoglobin levels that are 30 percent greater than women.

Food cooked in iron utensils are rich in iron, especially if the cooking process is long. Beans and roasts cooked in iron pots once made iron deficiencies rare, but now that ceramic and aluminum cooking utensils have largely replaced iron this is no longer a source. Natural food sources include apricots, peaches, bananas, molasses, prunes, raisins, and brewer's yeast. Among vegetables, spinach, beet and turnip greens, and alfalfa are good sources.

Vitamin C aids in absorption of iron. A product that contains iron plus vitamin C is therefore ideal, if you have an iron deficiency. Incidentally, coffee and tea interfere with iron absorption. Elderly persons often lack sufficient gastric acid to absorb iron, and these persons are more prone to iron deficiency anemia. A superior product will contain iron in a naturally bound organic form, which is not only better tolerated, but more completely absorbed. Inorganic forms of iron, commonly used in most supplements and for "enriched" bread, destroys vitamin E as well as being harsh on the digestive system.

Since for most of us, especially males, and females past menopause, iron is a toxin to be avoided, you may want to get rid of the excess iron you have accumulated over the years. The easiest and most beneficial way is to donate blood perhaps three times a year. Another way is to undergo chelation therapy, since iron is readily removed by EDTA chelation.

Only 2 to 3 milligrams of copper are required daily, but the average diet supplies only about half this much. Copper is toxic in excess. Sufficient copper to meet minimum requirements apparently can be abosrbed through the skin from copper bracelets worn to ease arthritis, an effective treatment for some individuals. Copper plumbing also is a good source of copper, but may result in toxic levels of copper if the water supply is soft or is acidic. If your sinks have a green copper stain where water drips it is most probable that you have a problem with copper toxicity. A hair analysis for excess copper is advised. Chlorine in the water reacts with the copper pipes to produce copper chloride. Copper is necessary for iron absorption, and is usually found in foods that are rich in iron. Copper absorption is blocked by excess zinc ingestion, but this usually is not a problem if less than 45 milligrams of zinc is taken supplementally.

Copper and zinc are both necessary to convert thyroxin (T4)

to tri-iodothyroxine (T3), the active form of the hormone. Therefore a deficiency of both minerals can produce hypothyroidism. It should be noted that the T3 and T4 levels in the blood can be entirely normal, and cellular levels of T3 be low because of copper and zinc deficiencies.

Since copper is necessary for production of RNA, healing cannot occur without it. Hair color is also dependent on copper. Drugs which contain copper chelates are potent anti-ulcer formulas. This is particularly interesting since aspirin removes copper from the stomach lining and transports it to the site of inflammation. Aspirin chelated with copper not only will not cause stomach ulcers, but will actually promote the healing of ulcers! Copper dependent diabetes has been proven.

Unfortunately, ionized copper has the same problem that is associated with ionized iron: production of free radicals. Therefore, you should not take copper supplements unless you have a documented deficiency. Two adequate tests are a hair analysis by a reputable laboratory, or an erythrocyte copper determination.

Manganese is a necessary mineral, but the RDA is unknown. Toxicity studies would suggest 20 milligrams daily as a reasonable supplement. It is known to be important in metabolism of carbohydrates, fat, and proteins, as well as RNA synthesis. In combination with choline (found in lecithin), it aids fat digestion and use. Manganese is also necessary for reproduction and the production of milk.

Manganese potentiates the effects of vitamin C, being essential in a reaction in which manganese is a co-factor with vitamin C. Even more importantly, manganese is a key element in the enzyme superoxide dismutase (SOD), one of the key enzymes necessary to neutralize free radicals. Superoxide dismutase is the fifth most common protein in the human body. Longevity is directly related to the amount of SOD within the body.

In 1982, I discovered that some patients with open angle glaucoma reverted to normal when 40 milligrams of manganese was added to the diet daily. It is effective only after about six weeks, and for some persons is effective at half that dose. Only about half my patients with open angle glaucoma have responded to manganese. Interestingly, vitamin A has recently (*Glaucoma,* December, 1982) been shown to be deficient in persons with glaucoma, and vitamin A is essential for protein synthesis. Since RNA is essential in the mechanism of protein synthesis, and RNA cannot be made without manganese, the two may be acting at the same point. We find the same type of relationship with zinc, because you cannot use your vitamin A without zinc.

Manganese is found in green leafy vegetables, blueberries, citrus, bran, peas, and seaweed. Wheat germ is probably the richest source. Deficiency symptoms include poor growth, sterility and impotence, poor equilibrium (due to middle ear problems), asthma, and myasthenia gravis. Manganese deficiency also results in abnormal development of bone and cartilage, and degeneration of the vertebral discs. Thus, chronic back pain can be a symptom of manganese deficiency. Other reported signs of manganese deficiency include epilepsy and diabetes. There has been one report of a diabetic who did not respond to insulin, but recovered with manganese supplements. Manganese is essential for the synthesis of insulin. Along this line, it is of interest that alfalfa tea is a folk remedy for diabetes, and alfalfa is a potent source of manganese. Blueberries, a good source of manganese, also tends to improve blood sugar levels.

Manganese is a calcium channel blocker, and just as potent as the recently introduced calcium channel blockers in controlling hypertension. Unfortunately, it is poorly absorbed and competes with other essential minerals.

Another mineral essential for healing is zinc, recently become popular and now added to virtually all supplements. Zinc is needed in about 15 milligrans per day, with more needed during times of stress. Toxic doses are possible. Daily supplementation of up to 45 milligrams is safe.

Zinc is essential for formation of both RNA and DNA, so healing and reproduction are impossible without zinc. Zinc is intimately involved with about seventy metabolic processes, including the synthesis of insulin, so that it is absolutely essential to life. Your body cannot use vitamin A without zinc. Again, this may be tied in with RNA synthesis, along with manganese. In addition to the expected effects of zinc deficiency (poor wound healing, poor skin and hair health, loss of the senses of taste and smell), zinc deficiency is associated with atherosclerosis.

In 1979, I accidentally discovered that 20 milligrams of zinc daily would reverse cataracts in many patients. My success rate using zinc along with vitamins has been about 67 percent. Salmon fed a zinc deficient diet develop cataracts. So do other animals. Incidentally, the lime added to soil to control pH is generally limestone from which the zinc has been removed.

Recent studies have shown that 85 percent of persons admitted to the intensive care units in both Boston and Atlanta were zinc deficient. Those most severely deficient generally died, most of those with mild or no deficiencies recovered. Since zinc deficiencies are common, the wise man will supplement his diet with zinc. Again, select a chelated product such as zinc picolinate or zinc orotate, which is readily used by the body.

Zinc present in seeds cannot be used by the body, unless the seeds have been sprouted or fermented. Other food sources are milk, eggs, onion, oysters, nuts, and green leafy vegetables. Note, however, that many soils are zinc deficient, and zinc is not commonly added to soil unless the farmer practices organic gardening. Organic mulch is generally rich in zinc. Of course, you don't eat the mulch, you feed it to your plants.

A friend asked me why mulch is effective in adding minerals to the soil, if the mulch was probably raised on mineral deficient soil. A good question. Obviously mulch from plants raised on rich soil would be superior. Even better would be a mulch of kelp or seaweed. But even though not ideal, the plants will contain small amounts of whatever minerals were present, since all life tends to concentrate the elements found in its environment. Eventually, by adding large amounts of mulch to your garden a healthy soil can be produced. Quicker results are obtained by also using products such as green sand and mineral rock.

Anytime you discover that a mineral or vitamin is essential for either RNA or DNA synthesis, a deficiency of that element can produce almost any effect. DNA is the basic genetic material, and no cell can reproduce without new DNA. Obviously, healing cannot occur without DNA. Proteins and enzymes (which are proteins) are made by instructions given by DNA through RNA. Thus any substance that is needed for RNA synthesis will affect virtually all metabolic processes. Memory requires RNA, so intelligence and learning will be affected by anything that limits RNA. Zinc is involved in *both* RNA and DNA synthesis. That is why zinc is one of the most important elements. Everyone would be wise to supplement their diet with at least 15 milligrams per day, and up to 45 milligrams during periods of stress or illness.

Silicon is a mineral which comprises fully one quarter of the earth's crust; it is the major element in sand and clay, and it is the magic element of the computer age. It may also be the magic element for nutrition and health. Epidemiologic studies in Finland finally isolated silicon as being the major protective factor preventing heart disease. Silicon-poor diets *invariably* induce deformities in the bones and cartilage of laboratory animals. It has also been proven that the elasticity and impermeability of arteries is directly proportional to the amount of silicon in the blood.

Arteries have to be elastic in order to smooth out the pressure pulses of the heartbeats; and if arteries are too permeable (leaky), edema results. Autopsy studies show that atherosclerotic arteries contain fourteen times less silicon than healthy arteries.

Rats whose diets were supplemented with silicon fused broken bones much faster than those with diets without silicon added. Silicon is known to be necessary for bone formation, but has not been used in treatment of human bone diseases such as osteoporosis and Paget's Disease of the bone. Its high concentration in the cornea, sclera, and vitreous of the eye make it a logical experimental choice in treatment in diseases afflicting these tissues.

Presently, very little is known about the need for silicon, except that it is needed. The RDA is unknown. It is common in most vegetables and yeast products, but is largely removed by commercial processing. It is essential for strong bones, healthy hair, nails and teeth, as well as for disease resistance. Aging is more rapid when silicon is deficient. Silicon deficiency is present in all degenerative diseases such as atherosclerosis and arthritis, and these diseases respond to foods rich in silicon. A diet rich in vegetables and fruit should contain sufficient silicon, and especially if the peelings are eaten. Research in this area is becoming active, and answers should be available in the not too distant future. It would be most surprising if we did not have a major role for such a common element. The major food sources are bran and alfalfa. Since processed foods have been stripped of bran, and alfalfa is not a common human food unless you are a health food nut (I am), what are the other sources of silicon? Pectin is, but we consume much less fruit today than a few decades ago. Yeast is a good source, and so also are beer and wine. All dietary fibers are good sources of silicon. But this does not include processed fiber additives such as cellulose, commonly added to some brands of high fiber bread. "Willard water," claimed to be effective in treatment of arthritis and other degenerative diseases, is made with sodium meta silicate and is thus a good source of silicon.

To understand why silicon is so beneficial, it should be noted that atoms within a molecule do not just sit there, but fairly freely exchange with other atoms similar in atomic size and electron configuration. Silicon is very similar to carbon, one of the principle atoms in living tissues, and will quickly replace carbon in bone, tendons, ligaments and other carbon molecules. Once silicon replaces carbon in connective tissue, as the tissue which literally holds us together is called, the resulting tissue is much stronger than it was previously. Also, silicon is bound more strongly than carbon, and will tend to displace carbon in body tissues. The siliconized molecule is much more resistant to degradation than before. Incidentally, silicon is highly concentrated in healthy synovial fluid, the fluid that lubricates bone joints. It looks as though God invented silicon lubricants before we did.

Since crude fiber is our major source of silicon, how can we tell that we have enough fiber in the diet? Dr. Bassler says that when the diet has enough fiber, the stool floats and is about 25 centimeters long.

Since most of us cannot get excited about atherosclerosis until we enter the coronary unit at the local hospital, perhaps it should be pointed out that the wrinkles and baggy skin due to lack of elastic tissue may be due in turn to silicon deficiency. It is entirely possible that all degenerative diseases are in part due to silicon deficiency. Certainly, silicon-rich collagen is less susceptible to oxidation by free radicals. The final word on silicon is yet to be said. In the meantime, pass the alfalfa, please.

Vanadium has not yet been proven to be an essential element for human health, but has been proven essential in two species of animals. Vanadium appears to be essential for growth and fat metabolism. A deficiency results in increased blood cholesterol and triglyceride levels. Supplementation with only a few milligrams of vanadium daily results in dramatic reductions in blood cholesterol levels. In areas where the soil is rich in vanadium, both heart and vascular disease is practically non-existent. Vanadium is similar to chromium, and an excess of vanadium (along with a deficiency of chromium and selenium) may cause cataracts. For those who consider the use of vanadium supplements as being far-fetched, consider that the 1958 edition of the *Archives of Internal Medicine* (101:685-689) recommends use of vanadium in the treatment of atherosclerosis. It seems we keep rediscovering the wheel.

Vanadium is very toxic, similar to arsenic in toxicity. Estimates of safe daily ingestion range from 100 micrograms to several milligrams. A compromise dose might be 500 micrograms daily, with frequent hair analysis to avoid overdosage.

Tin is another mineral essential for growth, but probably taken in adequate quantities due to its use in tin cans. Very little else is known about tin requirements. As tin cans become less common, modest supplementation should be considered.

XXII.
The Trace Elements

The trace elements are those elements which are required in microgram quantities. To get an idea of how little that is, consider that a level teaspoon could hold about 4,500,000 micrograms of salt. The dot at the end of this sentence weighs several micrograms.

The trace elements with known importance are selenium, lithium, cobalt, molybdenum, chromium, fluorine and iodine. Other trace elements which probably are important, but whose purpose is far from clear include boron and nickel. Some of these elements are present in the body, but may not actually be serving any useful purpose. All metals possess strong electrical force fields, and have a physical size peculiar to that metallic ion; the combination of size and electrical force field makes a metallic ion like a magic key which unlocks specific metabolic processes. In the case of lithium and bromine, they seem to slow down normal processes by interfering with other ions. This slowing down of activity has a tranquilizing effect that can be useful in selected cases. In excess, all of the minor and trace elements are very toxic. Interestingly, the maximum beneficial level of many of the trace elements is very close to the toxic levels.

The higher up the food chain, the more the trace elements are concentrated; assuming, of course, they are present in the environment. By intensively farming with chemical fertilizers, we have interfered with the food chains and reduced the trace element levels in our vegetables. Organic gardening methods, in which leaves and other organic matter is used for mulch and fertilizer, will eventually restore the soil to full health and vitality. Much of our farmland is now sterile and almost dead through decades of abuse. Dig for worms and you will find none where they thrived only two decades ago. This is not a tragedy: it is an ecological disaster.

Iodine was one of the first trace minerals discovered, partially because a deficiency in iodine results in goiter, which is very obvious. Iodine is the active element in thyroxin, a hormone made by the thyroid gland. When iodine is deficient, the thyroid gland swells immensely, producing a goiter. Thyroid hormone regulates the metabolic rate, and therefore affects almost everything we do.

We need about 150 micrograms of iodine daily. This is easily obtained through proper diet, and supplementation is not necessary. The sea is the best source of iodine, and people living near the oceans do not develop a deficiency because their diet contains ample seafoods. Rich sources include kelp, seaweed, seafoods, Spirulina, sea salt, and iodized salt. Iodine will pass through the skin, so tincture of iodine applied to the skin will also supply a hefty dose of iodine. Iodine was added to salt some decades ago in an effective effort to eliminate goiter. If the soil contains iodine, Swiss chard, turnip greens, garlic, water cress, pineapple, pears, artichokes, and citrus are good sources. Artichokes and pineapple grow in areas that get a lot of salt ocean spray, so they are always good sources.

With a mineral so important as iodine, there should be some natural mechanism for moving iodine inland. There is. Micro-organisms living in the ocean produce a compound called methyl iodine, which quickly disperses as a gas into the atmosphere, and is carried with the clouds to be deposited in the soil with the rains. The fact that goiter did not occur in everyone is ample evidence of the effectiveness of this mechanism. The presence of this mechanism has been used as one piece of evidence that our planet is a living organism. (This evidence is presented in the book, *Gaia*, by J. E Lovelock, published by the Oxford University Press. I heartily recommend it to your inquiry.)

Radioactive iodine is a natural part of fallout from nuclear explosions. This radioactive iodine is dispersed by the winds, and is rapidly picked up by the thyroid gland. In high doses, such as would occur after a nuclear war, many would suffer irreparable damage to their thyroid glands, and some would later develop cancer of the thyroid gland. It has been advised that everyone keep a supply of supersaturated potassium iodide available to take immediately if such a disaster occurs, since a few drops of this would saturate the thyroid gland, and prevent the radioactive iodine from being absorbed. A few ounces will provide sufficient protection for an entire family.

Fluorine was discovered to be important by epidemiologic studies that demonstrated that dental caries (decay) was rare in areas where the water supplies had natural levels of fluoride. In excess, fluoride causes mottled teeth, and is toxic. In proper quantities, it greatly strengthens teeth and bone. The amount of fluorine needed daily is unknown.

A lot of controversy has been made about the adding of fluoride to the water supplies, with reasons for opposition ranging from the fact that it smacks of socialized medicine, to the fact that fluorine is poison. The facts belie the critics. True, fluorine is poison, but fluorine is not used: what is used is a salt of fluorine which is non-toxic in the quantities used. Like all of the elements, it is poisonous in excess, but greatly beneficial in proper quantities. Even an overdose of water is lethal.

More attention should be paid to the use of chlorine, which is very poisonous and may actually be a major cause of atherosclerosis. Chlorine gas is added to our water supplies to oxidize the bacteria and organic wastes in the water. It is a very effective poison and does its job very well. But it is also very poisonous to us. No studies have ever been done to prove the safety of chlorine. Studies have been done proving that chlorinated water supplies will cause atherosclerosis in animals (chickens). An oxidant, chlorine destroys antioxidant vitamins such as vitamin C and E, and is a potent producer of free radicals. In combination with sodium, chlorine is essential. But what we need is chloride ions, not chlorine gas.

I have diverted thus far in order to show that the ion (fluoride) is not toxic like the pure substance (fluorine). The opposition to the addition of fluoride to the water supply has no justification. I would suggest that perhaps other trace elements could also be effectively added to the water supply, or to fertilizers so that our vegetables would naturally contain them. The quantities needed to be added to the water supply would be very minimal, but would have to be adjusted to reflect regional differences. Another approach might be to add them to salt just as we add iodine now. China is using this approach for selenium supplementation. The disadvantage of socialized supplementation is seen in the case of iron, where we are now getting toxic amounts of that essential element. Should we trust a government that has given us kudzu, the multiflora rose, and the IRS?

Chromium is a trace element which only recently has become recognized as essential. Supplementation with 100 to 200 micrograms daily is recommended.

Chromium is part of several enzymes and hormones. It is a co-factor with insulin, and as such is essential for regulation of blood sugar. A recent article in the JAMA (June, 1982) confirmed that chromium will normalize both hypoglycemia, and hyperglycemia. The dosage used was 200 micrograms per day. It is especially interesting that white sugar causes a loss of chromium, since the high consumption of white sugar (over 100 pounds per person per year!) has been associated with both an increase in abnormal glucose metabolism and an increase in heart disease. One study in London concluded that persons who consume over 120 pounds of white sugar per year are fifteen times more likely to have coronary disease, compared to persons who consume less than sixty pounds of white sugar per year. You may argue that you don't buy more than ten pounds per month, so your family could not be consuming that much sugar. I invite you to go to your cupboard and look at the list of ingredients for virtually everything from catsup to pork and beans. Sugar and salt are present as major ingredients in almost all processed foods.

How does this tie into chromium? Remember, white sugar causes the loss of chromium, moving chromium across cell membranes into the blood where it is transported to the kidneys and excreted. Chromium is also necessary for insulin to be able to move glucose into cells. And chromium is necessary for the synthesis of heart protein (muscle), and is important in cholesterol metabolism. Chromium deficiency is probably why white sugar is implicated in diabetes, hypoglycemia, heart disease, and athero-sclerosis. If sugar is the culprit, why is raw sugar not also guilty? The answer is as plain as the nose on your face: raw sugar is an excellent source of chromium! Again, in his wisdom, our Father provided the chromium we need along with the sugar which requires chromium for its efficient use.

Chromium is naturally present in hard water (but is not present in the water of the southeastern U.S.), whole grains, mushrooms, liver, brewer's yeast, raw sugar and molasses. It is also present in wine and beer if they are fermented in stainless steel vats, since stainless steel is made with chromium. This may explain why alcoholics do not develop atherosclerosis nor heart disease. (They do develop cirrhosis of the liver, which is worse. I am not advocating alcoholic beverages as a source of chromium!) The proper daily allowance of chromium is about 200 micrograms daily.

Glucose Tolerance Factor is a complex of chromium with niacin and three amino acids. In this form, chromium acts more like a hormone than an element, and can substitute for insulin in selected individuals. GTF can be produced by growing yeast in chromium rich broth, and is effective when taken orally. Diabetics appear to be unable to effectively synthesize GTF from chromium, and should take their chromium as GTF. However, trivalent chromium is effective in regulating blood sugar in clinical hyper- and hypo-glycemia in nondiabetics.

Chromium deficiency is associated with coronary disease and atherosclerosis, as well as with elevated cholesterol levels. Regression of atherosclerotic plaques has been demonstrated in animals whose diet contained supplemental chromium. Reversal of atherosclerosis has not been proven in man, but the association of chromium deficiency with atherosclerosis has been proven.

Since chromium and iron bind to the same blood protein, an excess of iron will result in a loss of chromium through the kidneys. This may be why an iron excess is associated with adult onset diabetes.

Molybdenum is essential, and is involved in carbohydrate metabolism. The quantity of molybdenum needed is unknown, but toxicity studies would suggest that as much as 20 milligrams daily are needed. The official RDA is between 150 and 500 micrograms daily. Fortunately, molybdenum is found in whole cereals, especially brown rice, buckwheat, and milet. It is also present in brewer's yeast and legumes (peas, alfalfa). Deficiencies are associated with cancer of the esophagus and gouty arthritis. The element seems to protect against tooth decay. Molybdenum is the key element in three enzymes, involved with fat oxidation and purine metabolism.

Molybdenum is protective against copper poisoning, which is almost definitely a problem if your plumbing is copper. However, I am not advising your taking molybdenum to correct a copper toxicity problem, as there are simply no answers at the present time. Molybdenum metabolism and requirements would be a fertile area for research, and should be investigated immediately so that crucial questions might be answered. We need to know how much is optimum, and whether our diet is providing it.

Cobalt is the metal ion present in vitamin B12. Actually, if cobalt were present in the diet, we would be able to synthesize vitamin B12, so that it is a vitamin in a relative sense only. Probably only about 1 microgram daily is needed. Cobalt would be present in liver, and in all green leafy vegetables, if the cobalt were in the soil. A big *if.*

Lithium is a micro-nutrient which may not be needed by everyone. It is somehow involved in sodium metabolism, and is used in therapy of schizophrenia and depression. This benefit may be a function of its interference with normal patterns rather than a usual function of lithium. People are different, and our metabolic needs vary also. I most certainly am not recommending routine lithium supplements.

Selenium is proving to be extremely important as a trace element. It is an antioxidant, and works parallel to vitamin E. Both potentiate the effects of the other. Selenium is also part of the enzyme glutathione peroxidase, essential in the regeneration of vitamin C after it has been oxidized by tocoperol quinone (see chapter on free radicals). Toxicity studies would indicate that between 50 and 500 micrograms daily would be a proper dosage for supplementation. Up to 2000 micrograms is safe, whereas 3000 micrograms may be toxic. Dairy products are excellent sources of selenium, with a glass of milk supplying fully 100 micrograms, depending on the source of milk. This may be rather constant since cattle are commonly fed mineral salts. Some areas of North America have volcanic soils rich in selenium and persons living in those areas do not need additional selenium. Nebraska is a prime example.

As an antioxidant, selenium has been accepted as important in preventing cancer by the National Academy of Sciences. In general, the more selenium in the diet, the less likely for cancer to develop. Since aging is primarily an oxidation process, selenium deficiencies are associated with premature aging. Whether adequate doses of the antioxidants will prevent aging in humans is unknown, but certainly this approach has been proven to work in animals. I personally view aging as a disease state, and consider the normal cycle being to live a vigorous life without aging until the genetic clock shuts us down at about 120 years of age. Heart disease is usually associated with selenium deficiencies, and both selenium and vitamin E have been effectively used in treatment of angina pectoris. A disease with symptoms similar to congestive heart disease has been proven to be due to selenium deficiency. The disease is so common among children in China that the Chinese are now adding selenium to table salt just as we add iodine here.

Selenium compounds are effectively used to treat dandruff. Interestingly, patients using such shampoos find that seborrhea elsewhere on their body also clears up, which is an indication that selenium salts pass through the skin. (I am aware of one patient who absorbed toxic amounts of selenium from taking whole body shampoos with a selenium product.) It is also probable that they are actually treating a selenium deficiency. In my own situation, I have had severe dandruff for many years. This has totally disappeared with the past year since I have been taking 50 micrograms of selenium daily. (I now take 1000 micrograms daily.)

Other vitamins or minerals may also have been beneficial. I no longer use anti-dandruff shampoos of any kind.

Selenium is also important for the proper function of the immune system, and thus resistance to disease, and is more effective when used in conjunction with vitamin E.

I had discovered in 1981 that vitamin E improved the vision of many of my patients with reduced vision without obvious cause. Some cataracts also cleared somewhat with the addition of vitamin E to the treatment. Later, I read that nutrition scientists had discovered that selenium was the metal ion active in the enzyme system glutathione peroxidase. Since this enzyme system is one of the ones which becomes less active during the development of cataracts, and since selenium and vitamin E practically substitute for each other, the tie-in became obvious. More recently, it has been proven that vitamin E will prevent and reverse diabetic cataracts. It should also be obvious why I now include both vitamin E and selenium in the treatment of all cataracts and vision disturbances. More recently, the National Institutes of Health has proven vitamin E to be essential for retinal function, thus it is necessary for vision. I predict that selenium will also prove necessary for vision.

An excellent source of selenium, especially when many mineral deficiencies exist, is Body Toddy™. Before taking over two ounces per day you should obtain a hair analysis from a reputable lab. An hair analysis kit may be obtained from Bio-Zoe, Inc., P.O. Box 49, Waynesville, NC 28786-0049.

In 1986, germanium had become the Cinderella element. Used generously in Japan, it is claimed to be virtually non-toxic and to do everything from reversing aging to curing cancer. In any case, it is rather expensive.

The preferred form is Bis-Beta-Carboxy-ethyl-Germanium sesquioxide, trade named GE-132. It is water soluble, and remains in the body less than 24 hours. It enhances interferon production and boosts the immune system. Its anti-tumor effects are currently being tested in clinical trials. Germanium's curative powers were discovered when it was found concentrated in healing herbs. A reasonable dose appears to be 50-150 milligrams three times daily. GE-132 seems to work by increasing cellular oxygen availability.

Note: I have now found that 1000 mcg of selenium (from sea kelp) daily for 4-10 months is necessary to restore adequate body levels.

XXIII.
Synthetic
Antioxidants

In the chapters on free radical pathology and a sane approach to it, several natural vitamins and elements involved in the neutralization of free radicals were mentioned. These include: beta carotene, vitamin E, vitamin C, riboflavin, niacin, selenium, manganese, and zinc. Additionally involved are copper and iron, but these also can catalyse free radical production in excess. Several enzyme systems are involved, but they are synthesized internally given adequate amounts of essential amino acids (from protein), and the elements mentioned above.

There are synthetic compounds that will effectively combat free radicals, and the peroxidation of fats. At present, there is some controversy about their use, with purists demanding the exclusion of all additives and manufacturers looking for a way to safely prolong the shelf life of their products. I think that it is safe to say that antioxidant compounds that prevent oxidation of food are beneficial to us, even when ingested. While they are preserving our food, they are also preserving us.

DMSO is a very potent synthetic solvent that has antioxidant properties. DMSO rapidly and effectively neutralizes free radicals, and is effective in reducing the severity of injuries when used promptly. It is especially effective for first and second degree burns, if applied immediately. It also seems effective in relieving the pain of bursitis. DMSO is being used experimentally in an attempt to reduce nervous system damage after injuries. DMSO is a useful addition to your medicine cabinet.

Hydergine (Sandoz) is an effective antioxidant that is most effective taken sublingually. A prescription is required. Although the FDA recommended dose is 3 milligrams a day, European doctors are using up to 9 milligrams daily. They find that by using Hydergine before surgery, or immediately upon arrival in the emergency room when there is brain injury or massive blood loss (blood loss results in anoxia, which produces a free radical crisis), results in remarkably increased survival rates and deceased morbidity. Hydergine will reduce the density of lipofuchsin deposits in the brain. These deposits normally increase with age, and are related to free radical pathology. Hydergine given to a mother in labor will reduce brain damage in her child. Persons going into a dangerous situation should seriously consider taking Hydergine before undertaking the task.

Santoquin (Monsanto) is a food antioxidant that has been used in animal feed for some years. Fed to expectant mice, the drug increases the life span of their offspring. Santoquin is very similar structurally to vitamin E. Santoquin will substitute for vitamin E in animals dependent on vitamin E. The recommended rate of application for animal feed is 125 ppm (0.01 percent). A rate of 0.5 percent increased the life span of mice 30-45 percent in a 1966 study.

BHT (butylated hydroxytoluene) is a powerful synthetic antioxidant, used extensively as a food preservative. Used as a food additive for animals in a life extension experiment (0.5 percent of food), it produced a 45 percent increase in life span, about the same as Santoquin. BHT powerfully inhibits viruses, including herpes and influenza, and has been successfully used in treatment of infections by these viruses. BHA is similar in effect to BHT. Adding a teaspoon of BHT to a quart of cooking oil immediately upon opening will prevent it from oxidizing. This dose is ten times the FDA recommended level, and I am passing this along for your interest. One teaspoon represents a 0.5 percent concentration of BHT in the oil. BHT is available from Eastman Chemical Products, Inc., Kingsport, Tennessee (1-800-251-0351). It is also available from Vitamin Research Products, Inc, 1961-D Old Middlefield Way, Mountain View, California 94043, (1-415-967-7770).

If you decide to use synthetic antioxidants in your own program of personal health, find a physician who will cooperate with you and perform the necessary laboratory tests to help keep you out of trouble. If you are going to ask for his assistance in your program, it is only fair that you agree in writing not to hold him responsible for the results. You will indeed be treading on uncharted soil. Your venture probably will be a success, but the risk is there. In any case, we know the risk of not venturing forth, and that risk is rather great.

XXIV.
Toxic Metals

All metals are toxic, taken in sufficient quantity. This includes those metals and elements proven essential for life. Those elements have been sufficiently covered in the chapters on the various elements.

This chapter is not intended to be all inclusive concerning all the other toxic elements (mainly heavy metals) that might be in the environment. Indeed, there are volumes written about this subject, and I am obviously not going to be able to condense this vast amount of knowledge into a few pages.

However, there are a few toxic elements to which we are exposed sufficiently for them to be a general health hazard, and it is these that I will address.

Most toxic elements are heavy metals: arsenic, cadmium, copper, lead, mercury, nickel, and such. Aluminum is not a heavy metal, but it most definitely is toxic and implicated in various degenerative diseases.

Lead is an industrial pollutant, but has been implicated in the fall of the Roman Empire. When Rome conquered Greece, the Greeks had already discovered that lead was poisonous, but the invading Romans were intrigued with beautiful Greek lead drinking vessels, and used Greek artisans to make these beautiful goblets for Roman aristocracy. Needless to say, why should a Greek slave ignore his masters wishes? Lead was also used to line fermenting vats for wine, and for plumbing in the homes of wealthier Roman citizens. Wine is acidic, and easily dissolves lead, forming lead acetate. Consumed, lead causes brain damage, dementia, and insanity. No wonder the Roman Empire fell, its leading citizens were poisoned with lead and incapable of leadership before they were 30 years of age. X-rays of the skeletons of Roman aristocracy have demonstrated sufficient lead to produce severe toxic effects.

In America, over 400,000 tons of industrial lead is released into the atmosphere annually. This settles into the soil, and is consumed. The Environmental Protection Agency yesterday announced that the health costs of leaded gasoline alone was five billion dollars a year. That, my dear reader, is your health they are talking about.

At least one in four Americans has toxic levels of lead within his body, clearly shown by a study involving over 38,000 citizens. Lead toxicity has as its early symptoms: headache, fatigue, muscle pains, decreased intelligence and memory, plus many other neurological deficiencies. You are very likely to suffer lead poisoning if you live in an urban area, or near major highways, or work in industries that use lead. Since paint once was lead based, the soil around old houses is saturated with lead. If you grow garden vegetables there, your vegetables will supply you with lead. In addition, you consume significant amounts of lead from the solder used in tin cans, and for copper plumbing. In fact, if you eat a lot of canned foods, you are exceeding toxic levels of lead from that source alone (as much as 106 micrograms of lead daily).

The problem of lead poisoning is genuine. Blood, urine, and hair analysis (the preferred test) can determine whether you have received toxic levels of lead already, almost a certainty. You can reduce your lead load by taking supplements of the various beneficial elements, which act to interfere with lead uptake, and vitamin C and B-complex which aid in the elimination of lead. In the end, avoiding lead exposure and EDTA chelation will prove necessary to get the lead out. The prudent reader will have the appropriate tests done and take action accordingly.

Cadmium is a toxin of the modern industrial revolution. Cadmium is used to plate metals to prevent rusting, including refrigerator ice trays (some of which are still being used). Cadmium is a principle metal in nickel cadmium batteries, which are an increasing source of groundwater cadmium as these batteries are thrown into the trash. Tobacco smoke, however, is the main source for most Americans.

Proven effects of cadmium toxicity include kidney damage (it interferes with zinc enzymes), hypertension, and cardiovascular disease. The only reliable test for cadmium levels is hair analysis.

A high calcium diet, plus other essential minerals will provide some protection against cadmium. Vitamin C aids in the excretion of cadmium. Zinc deficiency increases the effect of cadmium toxicity, so zinc supplements are indicated. Cadmium is removed by EDTA or 2-diaminocyclohexane disodium zinc tetra-acetate chelation therapy.

Mercury is also an industrial metal, and is used extensively in silver amalgams to fill dental cavities. It is very likely that you are carrying around a lot of mercury in your teeth. Mercury is used as a preservative for many medications, including eye and nose drops. Thimersol and merthiolate are mercury-based poisons used to kill bacteria. You are absorbing more mercury from this source than you can imagine.

Mercury is such an effective poison that it is applied to seed to prevent their rotting in the soil before germinating. Unfortunately, the plants take up this mercury and deliver it to your table. Mercury based fungicides are also sprayed freely on fruit to protect them from blight, but again, you consume the residues.

Symptoms of mercury poisoning include those common to the other heavy metals: neural damage and its ramifications, sensory loss (vision, hearing, taste, etc.), hypertension, and kidney damage. Hair analysis is the only accurate way to determine the extent of chronic mercury poisoning. Fortunately, selenium is effective in binding mercury ions and preventing their absorption. Chelation is effective in removing mercury from the body.

The mention of dental fillings as a source of mercury may surprise you, as it did me. Supposedly, the mercury in dental fillings is bound and not released. This is simply not so. A few months ago, a fellow physician active in preventive medicine, Dr. Roy Kupsinel of Oviedo, Florida, proposed that he test mercury levels in my breath both before and after my chewing gum for ten minutes. The initial reading was low (ideally, it should have been zero), but after chewing gum for ten minutes, the levels of mercury vapor in my breath was many times accepted toxic levels. This physician claims that bizarre symptoms that recur after meals may be due to mercury poisoning released from dental amalgams. In fact, he has many case histories that substantiate his claim. I am aware of one case of intractable hypertension which proved to be due to mercury poisoning from dental amalgams. The solution is to have a hair analysis done, then have your silver amalgam fillings replaced with gold or ceramic fillings.

Unfortunately, the American Dental Association, which led the fight for preventive dentistry, denies that mercury amalgams are a danger to patients. They do warn dentists and dental assistants to take strong precautions against mercury exposure, however. You would be wise to do likewise.

Aluminum consumption is increasing, and along with this is increasing evidence that aluminum is a significant neurological poison. Aluminum has been linked to senile dementia (Alzheimer's disease), Parkinson's disease, and dialysis dementia. Aluminum binds to DNA (the stuff of life itself), deposits in the brain, and interferes with some body enzymes. Aluminum is excreted through the kidneys, but will be deposited in bone if kidney function is abnormal. The major source of aluminum in the diet is its use in baked goods (baking powder) and in antacid tablets and suspensions. Aluminum foil and cooking utensils are probably a minor source, except for foods requiring prolonged cooking. Patients undergoing renal dialysis are given massive doses of aluminum, and suffer severe aluminum toxicity as a result. This contention is well supported by autopsy studies. So far, there is apparently no adequate substitute for use of aluminum to bind the phosphorus in these patients, which is a matter of personal concern since my father is currently on dialysis.

On the basis of current knowledge, I believe that avoiding use of foods with aluminum additives is indicated. Alum (used in pickles) and baking powder are primary examples. Anti-perspirants also use aluminum salts as the active ingredient, and this is absorbed through the skin. The major source of aluminum is probably antacid medications, which I would strongly urge you to avoid. Magnesium antacids are equally effective, and also supply a modicum of magnesium. I see no problem with aluminum utensils, especially if they are coated with Teflon, and unless they are used for foods that require hours of preparation, such as stews or soups. Aluminum beverage cans may be a problem since acids will partially dissolve aluminum. Research in this area is urgently needed.

Hair analysis is a valid method of detecting aluminum loads within the body. Excess aluminum is readily excreted through healthy kidneys. Desferoxamine, an iron chelator, also effectively removes aluminum when taken orally. Fluoride binds and removes aluminum, and EDTA chelation is also effective.

Arsenic is also toxic, but readily excreted once the environ-mental load is removed. Hair analysis is an effective method of detecting arsenic toxicity.

It should be noted that hair analysis, performed by a reputable laboratory, is an accurate method of detecting toxic levels of these elements. Since hair analysis costs only about $45 to $75, depending upon the tests performed, it is a logical first step toward improved health. Hair analysis will also detect low (and high) levels of certain essential trace elements, such as chromium, copper, selenium, and zinc.

In view of the fact that you are very apt to have toxic manifestations of one or more of these elements, I strongly urge the reader to have a hair analysis performed on each member of his family, and proceed accordingly. Hair analysis kits may be obtained from Bio-Zoe, Inc., P.O. Box 49, Waynesville, NC 28786-0049.

XXV.
Suggested Supplementation

Included below is a table of my personal daily supplementation recommendations. Some items, such as phosphorus, are so richly supplied in the diet that no supplementation is recommended. Exposure of the skin to sunlight will provide enough of this vitamin D to offset any deficiency children may have. Vitamin D supplementation is so common in America that adults may be already getting toxic amounts.

There is a continuing argument about the relative advantages of natural versus synthetic vitamins. The only advantage of the natural vitamins is that they usually also contain other nutrients which may not have been identified yet. Silicon was one of these unknowns until very recently. It is highly likely that we do not have the answers for all of our nutritional needs, and until we do some discretion is in order. For example, synthetic vitamin C is not associated with bioflavinoids, the natural product *may* be, depending on the processor. If, however, bioflavinoids are added, the synthetic vitamin C is fully acceptable. The synthetic vitamins are almost always cheaper, and have a much less risk of allergic reactions. Unfortunately, many products promoted as 100 percent natural are mainly synthetic with a small amount of the natural vitamin added. Minerals generally are better absorbed and less toxic if they are chelated with an amino acid, as they would be in a natural source. Non-chelated iron, for example, will destroy vitamin E; chelated iron will not, unless you already have an excess amount of iron.

PROPOSED DAILY SUPPLEMENTATION FORMULA:

Vitamin A	10000	IU
Beta carotene	15000	IU (easily supplied by diet)
Vitamin D3	400	IU
Vitamin E	400	IU
Vitamin C	500	mg.
Bioflavinoids	100	mg.

B1 (thiamine)	40	mg.
B2 (riboflavin)	20	mg.
B6 (pyridoxine)	40	mg.
B12 (cyanocobalamine)	100	mcg.
Niacin	50	mg.
Niacinamid	50	mg.
Pantothenic Acid	200	mg.
Folic Acid	800	mcg.
Biotin	300	mcg.
Choline	90	mg.
Inositol	90	mg.
PABA	50	mg.
Calcium	500	mg.
Magnesium	500	mg.
Phosphorus*	0	mg.
Iron*	0	mg.
Iodine*	150	mcg.
Copper	2	mg..
Manganese	20	mg.
Zinc	20	mg.
Molybdenum	100	mcg.
Chromium (GTF)	200	mcg.
Selenium	300	mcg.
Vanadium	500	mcg.
Germanium	?	

Supplementation with as much as an additional gram of calcium, and half that much magnesium might prove useful for those with significant deficiencies. Silicon supplementation currently should be through natural foods: alfalfa, cabbage family, lettuce, onions, dark greens, kelp, comfrey, milk, unmilled cereal grains (rice, oats, wheat, barley), soybean meal, and pectin. The amount of silicon needed is well over a gram a day, easily supplied with an unprocessed diet. Silicon is especially important to growing children, and in adults to maintain bone and tissue strength.

Deliberately less than RDA because of excesses in current American diet. Iron and copper should be supplemented only if a deficiency is proven.

Note: The optimum RDA for Manganese, Molybdenum, Chromium, Selenium, and Vanadium has not been established. The suggested supplement is within published safety ranges.

XXVI.
Essential Fatty Acids

When fat is digested, it is broken down into glycerol and long chain fatty acids. Some of these fatty acids are essential building blocks used by the body to make cell membranes (cell walls) and certain hormonal substances. Perhaps the most important of these is prostacyclin I2 (PGI2) and prostocyclin I1 (PGI1).

Please bear with me while I try to untangle a rather complicated subject. In trying to make it understandable I may make a few errors of omission, but I believe the conclusions to be valid.

Cis-cis linoleic acid is a common essential fatty acid, richly found in most unprocessed vegetable oils. The body uses *cis-cis* linoleic acid to produce prostacyclin I1, which has some very useful properties. First, it is a vasodilator (thereby lowering blood pressure). Second, it blocks the conversion of aracidonic acid to thromboxane A2 (TXA2), a compound which promotes platelet clumping which is the precursor of a thrombus. A thrombus, of course, is the necessary first step in a myocardial infarction (heart attack) or stroke. The conversion of *cis-cis* linoleic acid to PGI1 requires an enzyme delta-6-desaturase (D6D) which converts the fatty acid to gamma lenolenic acid. D6D becomes deficient as we grow older, thereby reducing the production of gamma lenolenic acid. This latter acid is converted to PGI1 thru the action of zinc, niacin, and pyridoxine. Vitamin C and a moderate amount of alcohol helps the conversion. Evening primrose oil is not only a rich source of linoleic acid (72%), but also of gamma lenolenic acid (9%). Evening primrose oil thus might prove beneficial to older persons who cannot produce their own gamma lenolenic acid from *cis-cis* linoleic acid.

Arachidonic acid is used by the endothelium (lining) of blood vessels to produce PGI2, which as noted above prevents the agglutination of platelets. Unfortunately, platelets use the same fatty acid to produce thromboxane A2 (TXA2) which promotes platelet agglutination. Arachidonic acid is supplied mainly by meat in the diet. Fortunately, vitamin E permits the production of PGI2 while blocking the synthesis of TXA2. The oil of garlic also has this same property. Thus arachidonic acid is beneficial in the presence of adequate levels of vitamin E, but may promote the production of a thrombus (clot) if vitamin E is deficient. A practical application of this knowledge would be to always take supplemental vitamin E if you eat meat or cook with garlic.

A fatty acid richly found in fish oils, eicosapentaenoic acid (EPA), is converted to a different prostacyclin, PGI3, and another compound (TXA3) which retard the production of platelet clumps. As a result, people whose diet consists mainly of fish (e.g., Eskimos) have virtually no deaths due to myocardial infarctions. This approach is currently being tested at several research centers. EPA in sufficient quantities can be obtained by eating cold water ocean fish or trout three times weekly, or by taking two EPA capsules per meal. Incidentally, it appears that EPA is so effective in reducing blood triglyceride levels that it also reduces the need for insulin. Apparently, insulin is partially blocked by high blood triglyceride levels.

Dihomogamma lenolenic acid, a metabolic step between gamma lenolenic acid and PGI1 is being tested in England as a means of reducing platelet agglutination. Preliminary reports are encouraging. This compound can be synthesized and will probably become a useful therapeutic drug. It is not actually a nutrient, but a natural metabolic product in healthy young people.

Margarine is a modified fat product manufactured from vegetable oils. In the process of manufacture, two toxic compounds are produced. *Cis-cis* linoleic acid is converted to *trans-trans* linoleic acid (at least 47% conversion rate), a synthetic fatty acid which did not exist in human food until the invention of margarine in 1920. This synthetic fatty acid blocks the conversion of *cis-cis* linoleic acid to PGI1. PGI1, as we have seen, is a vasodilator and prevents platelet agglutination. In addition, the *trans-trans* linoleic acid substitutes for natural fatty acids as a building block for cell membranes, and results in defective cell membranes. A cell is able to function and live because of its healthy cell membrane. A cell with a defective membrane cannot function in a normal manner. Thus a defective cell membrane allows extracellular calcium and sodium to leak into the cell, and normal intracellular magnesium and potassium to leak out. The result is hypertension, wasted energy expended by the cell to stay alive, and reduced vitality. A cell half alive produces a body half alive.

Secondly, margarine contains lactones, ring shaped molecules produced when a long chain fatty acid is heated. These synthetic molecules block the activity of the enzyme, plasmin, whose function it is to dissolve platelet clots. Incidentally, this activity of lactones can be blocked by 60 milligrams of pyridoxine daily. (Onion and garlic oils also have fibrolytic activity.)

Thirdly, margarine shares with all unsaturated fats its ease of oxidation into lipid peroxidases, which are our major source of toxic free radicals. Free radicals, as mentioned earlier, increase the likelihood of thrombus formation (blood clots) and cancer.

Thus, margarine increases the possibility of thrombus formation by three mechanisms: interference with the conversion of *cis-cis* linoleic acid to PGI1, increased production of free radicals, and the reduction of thrombus lysis (breakup) due to the action of lactones. The incidence of myocardial infarctions is almost parallel to the consumption of margarine.

Support for this thesis comes from the fact that solid malignant tumors spread by attachment to platelet thrombi. In Japan, men smoke much more than men smoke in America, but without the high incidence of lung cancer. The Japanese do not consume margarine. The assumption is that without margarine, thrombus (clot) formation is less likely, and thus the tumor is not able to spread easily. A recent study from Australia demonstrated that sunbathers who consume margarine rather than butter are 700% more likely to develop malignant melanomas. That this effect is due to *trans-trans* linoleic acid is confirmed by the fact that European margarine, which is limited to 3% *trans-trans* linoleic acid, does not have the same toxicity as American margarines.

Alpha linoleic acid is another acid which reduces platelet agglutination. Alpha linoleic acid deficiency produces psychological changes, even psychosis. Beriberi patients were also alpha linoleic acid deficient, since white rice is devoid of this essential fatty acid. White flour also is devoid of this essential acid, which is richly found in whole wheat and rye breads. Food grade linseed oil and Evening Primrose oil are also excellent sources. Unless your diet contains freshly ground wheat or rye flour you are deficient in this essential fatty acid. The modern American diet is almost totally devoid of alpha linoleic acid. Incidentally, all the linseed oil pressed in the United States is manufactured by two manufacturers. High quality linseed oil, whether purchased in the paint store or health food store, is identical. One physician who has used both linseed oil and safflower oil with his patients says that the linseed oil is far more effective. He prescribes one teaspoon per day.

Cystoid macular edema, swelling of the back of the eye that is a common complication of cataract surgery, may be in part due to margarine toxicity, or essential fatty acid deficiency. I have one patient who developed cystoid macular edema a few months after his first operation, which cleared slowly over a period of several months with conventional therapy. A year later, I removed his second cataract, and within two months he again developed CME, this time in BOTH eyes. For a six month period I tried vitamins, steroids in high doses, and non-steroidal anti-inflammatory drugs, all to no avail. His vision remained stuck at 20/200: blind in both eyes. His distress was none less than my own. One day, inspiration hit me and I asked if he used margarine. Indeed he did, lots of it. I took him off margarine and had him begin with one tablespoon of safflower oil daily, which he obtained from the grocery store. Within two weeks he could see 20/25 in each eye. I now encourage all of my patients, especially those with macular disease or cardiovascular disease to stop using margarine and substitute butter. Butter is better.

In summary, the seed oil industry has produced a nationwide dietary deficiency in alpha and *cis-cis* linoleic acid, while introducing toxic *trans-trans* linoleic acid and lactones into the diet. In addition, processing increases the production of toxic free radicals. Finally, they have added insult to injury by removing for separate sale any vitamin E which would have protected us against some of these toxic products.

As an ophthalmologist, it is of interest to me that some cases of dry eye syndrome respond to treatment with essential fatty acids. In fact, some of my patients report improvement merely by switching from margarine to butter. Vitamin A, deficient in the diet of a majority of Americans, will also cure dry eye syndrome and keratitis sicca. I use cod liver oil capsules.

L-Carnitine, a vitamin-like substance found in meats, acts to transport fatty acids across cell membranes, where they are utilized. L-Carnitine rapidly lowers low density blood cholesterol (the bad kind) and increases high density blood cholesterol levels. Taken with Evening primrose oil, L-Carnitine is beneficial in lowering blood pressures, reducing thrombus formation, and in lowering harmful cholesterol levels. All of these benefits can be attributed to the effective use of essential fatty acids.

All seed products (wheat, rye, oats, sunflower, etc.) are rich sources of the essential fatty acids. Additionally, nuts such as walnut, pecan, hickory, and almonds, and fruit such as avocado are rich sources of these essential nutrients. Unfortunately, these unsaturated fats are oxidized quickly upon exposure to air and heat, as would occur upon pressing the oils or grinding flour. Thus, the essential fatty acids can easily be obtained by eating seed products whole, or by grinding your flour immediately before baking bread. This last suggestion may seem extreme, but was clearly proven over four decades ago and well documented in Dr. Price's book listed in the bibliography. Highly processed fats such as margarine and vegetable shortening should be totally avoided.

Essential fatty acids, especially when taken with L-Carnitine, seem to produce long-term moderate weight loss. The effect begins after about 6 weeks of daily supplementation.

They also seem to be beneficial in boosting immunity against cancer. One study in England reportedly had 75% of terminal cancer patients go into remission when put on six capsules of Evening primrose oil daily.

A sensible approach to essential fatty acid balance would be to include a handful of whole nuts in your daily diet. Black walnuts have a superior oil. A quarter avocado will also supply your daily ration of oil, as would a few slices of whole grain bread or a handful of seed, such as sunflower, sesame, or pumpkin. Ripe olives are another dietary source. Finally, you could take a teaspoon (5cc) of food grade linseed oil or a tablespoon (15cc) of safflower oil daily, either straight or mixed with vinegar and spices as a salad dressing. The most expensive option would be to take capsules of Evening Primrose oil. If you are over 45 and your triglycerides are up, the gamma lenolenic acid in Evening primrose oil is worth a try. Other sources of gamma lenolenic acid include black walnut oil, and black currant seed oil. Whatever your source of oil, L-Carnitine will make its use more efficient. With an adequate vitamin C intake we should be able to synthesize our own L-Carnitine, but it is also worth the try. Finally, protect yourself from the toxic effects of arachidonic acid found in meat by adding vitamin E to your supplement regimen. This will cause arachidonic acid to be metabolized into a beneficial substance, preventing thrombus formation, rather than a harmful one which promotes thrombus formation. Garlic appears to have the same beneficial effect.

XXVII.
A Safe and Sane Diet

Since the publication of the first edition of this book, many have asked for a recommended safe and sane diet. Actually, this is found already within this book, but there is a need to bring it all together in a sensible form. Another similar approach is in the book, *By-Passing ByPass* found in the recommended reading list.

First, some general rules. Eliminate to whatever degree possible white sugar and white flour products from your diet. Also eliminate, again so far as practical, fried foods, especially those fried in vegetable oils or vegetable shortening. If you do eat fried foods, fry them in either butter, PAM™ or animal fat, beef suet being ideal.

Second, consume as much as possible of your fruit and vegetables raw and unprocessed, eating the peelings whenever practical. Obviously, some foods cannot be eaten raw. Whenever vegetables are cooked, steaming or cooking in the microwave oven is preferred. Do not overcook. Properly cooked vegetables are crisp and crunchy, not mush. If water is used in the cooking, do not throw away the water, because with it you will throw away the essential water soluble vitamins and minerals. Save it and use it for soups, or drink it. The pot liquor left from cooking greens is delicious with cornbread, as any Southerner will tell you. After he has eaten his share.

Your diet should supply at least two generous servings per day of dark yellow, or dark green vegetables or fruit. Especially good are spinach, broccoli, kale, sweet potatoes, pumpkin, squash, peaches, apricots, cantaloupes, and watermelon. Each of these is an excellent source of beta carotene, proven to be effective in preventing cancer. The vegetable sources are not only cheaper than taking this essential nutrient by tablet, they also taste so much better.

Don't neglect fruit, and include at least two fruit per day in your diet. If you are trying to lose weight, increase that to four, preferably eaten before meals. Eat your fruit whole, peeling and all, and chew it.

Don't cut it up into tiny pieces unless you must. Chewing is an essential part of nutrition since it activates digestive enzymes in the stomach and intestine. Chewing also tends to suppress the appetite.

Include one serving from the cabbage family each day, either raw or cooked. These include cabbage, broccoli, and cauliflower. Foods of the cabbage family have been shown to suppress cancer development, although an excess will also suppress the thyroid gland.

In an ideal world you would grind your own mixed grains and bake your bread, as we do. Flour begins losing its nutritional value immediately upon milling, and should be baked into bread within 24 hours of milling. A classical proof of this is found in Dr. Price's book listed in the bibliography. But you do need to include grain products in the diet, and they should be mixed grains if at all possible. By mixing various types of grain a more complete protein is provided, which translates into better nutrition. Basically, eat two servings of seed foods daily. That is, foods that reproduce themselves: beans, corn, sunflower seed, wheat, barley, etc. Many seeds are better sprouted and used with a salad. Popular for this are mung beans and alfalfa. My wife sprouts wheat to include in the flour she has ground, and that produces a softer bread.

Eggs are good nutrition, and should not be neglected. Forget the bugaboo that they raise your blood cholesterol. Even six eggs a day will not affect your blood cholesterol if they are boiled, poached, or fried without breaking the yolk sac. This has been proven in controlled scientific studies. If you do fry them, use butter, animal fat, or PAM™. At least one egg per day is recommended. Two at breakfast would be even better. I do not recommend scrambled eggs or omelets, because the cooking process exposes the cholesterol in the yolk to oxygen and heat, and also increases the oxidation and absorption of oil. Eggs cooked in this manner have more fat, contain toxic oxidized cholesterol, and should be avoided. One or two per week probably do minimal harm, however.

In order to get your essential fatty acids you should include one of the following in your diet daily: a handful of seeds or nuts, a quarter of an avocado, a generous serving of cold water ocean fish (or trout), or a salad dressing made with fresh safflower oil. A generous serving of wheat germ will also suffice, and can be eaten as a cereal. If you cannot get this in your diet, then supplement with a tablespoon of safflower oil or a teaspoon of linseed oil, or four capsules of MaxEPA™ available through your health food store. Evening primrose oil may be superior, especially for those of us over forty.

You need less than one gram of protein per kilogram of body weight per day. For the average seventy kilogram male, that comes to only 45 grams per day. The excess will be converted to energy and, if not used, stored as fat. Excess protein puts a heavy burden on your kidneys, and results in hyptertension. Persons with kidney disease, especially, should restrict their protein intake. Three and one-half ounces of meat daily will more than supply your protein needs, and if you eat a mixture of grains and legumes (beans and peas) you do not need to eat meat. However, most of us will eat meat. Trim the fat from the meat before cooking; or in the case of poultry, remove the skin. Buy only the leanest, freshest hamburger, and cook it promptly. The mixture of blood, air, and fat found in hamburger is especially potent in forming deadly free radicals. Fish and poultry are probably preferred to beef or pork, but that is mainly because of the oils in fish, and the low fat in poultry (especially if you remove the skin). However, lean beef or pork should not be avoided: they are good, and good for you. In order to get the fish oils now shown to reduce the risk of heart attack and stroke, it is recommended that you eat fish about three times per week, and certainly no less often than once per week. Meats should be cooked by slow cooker, or by roasting or grilling. Slow cooking at low temperatures is preferred.

Vitamin A is the vitamin most likely to be deficient in the American diet, and at least 60% of us are deficient in this vitamin. Most can convert the vegetable sources of vitamin A (the beta carotenes found in dark green and yellow fruit and vegetables), but at least 20% cannot make that conversion. These must eat the animal form of vitamin A found in liver, eggs, and fish liver oils. A serving of liver once a week is ample.

Dairy products supply calcium and protein. Unfortunately, they also supply a lot of fat. In addition, homogenized milk is made by breaking fat particles down so small that they cannot come together again. This keeps the cream from separating and floating to the top. It also makes a more marketable product. Unfortunately, these micron sized fat droplets pass through the intestinal walls without being digested, and may be a cause of atherosclerosis. Skim milk, or unprocessed milk is recommended until this issue is settled. Hard cheeses, such as swiss or provalone, have less fat than the soft cheeses. In any case, a couple of servings of dairy products daily are recommended. An ideal form is yogurt, which has been shown to lower blood triglycerides and cholesterol levels, as well as restore normal bacteria flora to the gut.

Water is a nutrient, and you need at least eight glasses of it a day. Unfortunately, municipal water supplies must be treated with chlorine and other chemicals to kill deadly bacteria and protozoa. Realize that the water coming from your tap must be sufficiently poison to kill anything in it. You are expected to be superman and drink it without harm. Ask any tropical fish merchant, tap water will kill your fish. It will also kill earthworms, reduce vegetable production by one third if you irrigate with it, and produce atherosclerosis in chickens when they drink it instead of well water. Chlorinated water is probably a major cause of atherosclerosis in man.

I strongly recommend installation of a water purification system. An ideal system would include both a resin exchange bed and activated charcoal, as well as a steam distillation. Reverse osmosis is also a good system. Each approach has its advantages. For further information write Bio-Zoe, Inc., Waynesville, NC 28786-0049. A good system can be installed for less than $1,000. The Rockland Water catalyst system appears good also, and will be useful even if you have well or spring water. This system adds electrons to water, thereby making it wetter. Catalyst activated water may be more effective in aiding absorption of minerals and for digestion. It is certainly beneficial when used for irrigation of plants. As a plus, it removes deposits from inside your home plumbing.

The average American diet gets 45% of its calories from fat, and 30% from white sugar. Much of the rest comes from white flour products. Meat supplies about 20% of our calories. The ideal diet should get about 25% of its calories from fat, preferably from sources mentioned above plus butter. None should come from margarine or hydrogenated fats. In other words, we need to eliminate half the fat from our diet. None of our calories should be coming from white sugar, or high sugar products such as carbonated beverages, confections, or the like. Fructose seems to be okay, as are raw sugar and molasses.

If you follow the guidelines in this chapter, plus supplement as needed to remineralize your body and supply those vitamins needed optimally in greater quantity, you will enjoy much improved health. Fiber, not mentioned in this chapter, will come automatically with this diet. If you need extra fiber, there are excellent fiber products on the market that can be eaten alone or added to your cooking.

Mineral deficiencies will occur even with this diet, primarily due to our severely deficient soils. A mineral supplement is strongly recommended. Most ideal will be a product such as Body Toddy™, taken one or two ounces per day. Although this product seems expensive, it is far, far less expensive than obtaining the same minerals in tablet form. A hair analysis obtained through Bio-Zoe, Inc., Waynesville, NC 28786-0049 will help you determine how severe your deficiency is, and how to correct it quickly. Obviously, I believe at least modest vitamin supplementation is prudent.

XXVIII.
The Miracle Supplements

The title "miracle" is used because the supplements discussed here often have effects so dramatic that they appear to be miraculous. They are naturally present in certain foods, and can be synthesized by the healthy individual. Therefore they are not vitamins in the strict sense of the word. However, like lecithin they seem to be produced in less than adequate amounts, and supplementation appears beneficial. More importantly, these compounds are totally non-toxic in even massive doses.

The first of these compounds to be discussed is *N,N Dimethylglycine (DMG)*, a naturally occurring metabolite. Strictly speaking, it is an intermediary metabolite, meaning that it is rapidly metabolized into other compounds. In the process, it makes the production of energy more efficient. Initial research in Europe and the USSR identified the compound Pangamic acid as vitamin B15. Most of their research refers to this compound as the active component, although later analyses have shown that the mixtures being tested contained free DMG as well. In any case, this use of an impure mixture led to decades of confusion in the scientific community. The American FDA was sufficiently convinced that Pangamic acid was not a vitamin that products labeled vitamin B15 are apt to be seized as fraudulent. Although Pangamic acid is metabolized within the body to DMG, it is not the most efficient way to obtain its benefits.

What is N,N Dimethylglycine? It is the amino acid glycine (part of all proteins) to which two methyl groups (-CH3) have been attached to the nitrogen atom. It acts as a methyl donor in our bodies, thereby causing desirable chemical reactions to proceed more smoothly. DMG is naturally found in many foods, but at a low levels. DMG acts like a catalyst in that it speeds certain chemical reactions, but is not a catalyst since it is destroyed in the reaction (it returns to glycine). We normally produce DMG in the catabolism (breaking down) of betaine and choline. Betaine itself can be synthesized from choline, which in turn is part of the lecithin molecule. This series of events may in part explain why lecithin is beneficial to many.

In any case, N,N Dimethylglycine is quickly broken down or metabolized in the liver to Sarcosine (mono-methylglycine) by the removal of one methyl group. This chemical reaction is catalyzed by iron and FAD (derived from riboflavin), and releases one molecule of hydrogen peroxide, which in turn provides extra oxygen at the cellular level. This reaction occurs primarily in the mitochondria of the liver. The removal of the second methyl group produces glycine and again is catalyzed by iron and FAD, again releasing one molecule of hydrogen peroxide at the cellular level. Thus DMG provides two single carbon units (methyl groups) and two molecules of hydrogen peroxide. The hydrogen peroxide provides needed oxygen at the cellular level, allowing for increased work without a buildup of lactic acid. Thus the use of DMG can delay fatigue during exercise, and also benefit tissues starved for oxygen such as the heart during angina. European and Soviet physicians use DMG extensively in treatment of cardiac conditions, and claim that it is extremely effective.

The two methyl groups removed are also extremely important. They are used to transform homocysteine (an amino acid) to the essential amino acid methionine. Methionine, as you may recall, is typically deficient in soybean protein, but is generally plentiful in other vegetable proteins. An essential amino acid is one we cannot produce ourselves, and therefore must be in the diet. With DMG, methionine ceases to be an essential amino acid. Other factors necessary for this reaction to occur are folic acid, riboflavin (as FAD), niacin (as NAD), vitamin B12, and Coenzyme Q10. Methionine is in turn used to produce another compound used throughout the body as a methyl donor.

The glycine that remains after removal of the two methyl groups is used to produce phosphocreatine, a high energy phosphate molecule used for energy in muscle and nerve tissue. Thus DMG is metabolized into several useful products that provide energy, oxygen, and methyl groups. DMG therefore beneficially affects every cell in the body.

DMG is very effectively absorbed through the intestinal tract and oral cavity. It is rapidly metabolized by the liver. Since any DMG absorbed through the intestines will pass first through the liver (and be instantly metabolized), it should be taken sublingually (under the tongue) to prolong the beneficial effect (which may be noted within twenty minutes). Even very large doses of DMG do not show up appreciably in the urine, again evidence that it is quickly metabolized and taken up into the tissues. Since none of the end products of DMG are toxic (all are beneficial), and since DMG is rapidly metabolized into these beneficial products, DMG is totally non-toxic. Well, not totally. The LD_{50} of DMG (as the hydrochloride salt) is 7.4 grams per kilogram of body weight. Since a standard tablet supplies 125 milligrams, by extrapolation it would take over 4,144 tablets in a single dose to be lethal to 50 percent of average 70 kilogram males. At current prices, that dose would cost $1,167.23, and would take impossibly long to swallow. A toxic dose is practically impossible in humans, especially since one would have to drink as much as fifty liters of water (in itself a lethal dose) to swallow these pills. In rats, ingestion of ten percent of the LD_{50} daily for two years produced no toxic effect, demonstrating its long-term safety.

DMG is hypoallergenic and non-mutagenic. That means that it does not produce allergic reactions, and does not increase the risk of cancer. The single report in the literature concluding a possible mutagenic effect has been proven to be in error by two independent laboratories. It has been used by thousands of clinicians and doctors for over a decade without adverse or negative side effects. Currently, the only pure form of N,N Dimethylglycine is manufactured by DaVinci Laboratories, under their U.S. patent #4,631,189. Nutritional factors that enhance the benefits of DMG include vitamins B2 (riboflavin), B6 (pyridoxine), B12 (cyanocobalamine), Niacinamide, Folic acid, Choline (part of lecithin), Betaine, iron, and magnesium.

Dimethylglycine has been proven at two universities to enhance both arms of the immune system, and to reduce susceptibility to cancer. DMG has been shown to enhance antibody production (T-cell proliferation and interferon production) by 400 percent. Since deterioration of the immune system is part of aging, it has been conjectured that DMG might be useful in slowing the aging process. AIDS, of course, is an immune deficiency disease. Boosting the immune system with DMG might prove very useful for those susceptible to infection, and for all of us during the influenza season. (Studies at Clemson University suggest its value in preventing influenza infections.) DMG also enhances exercise tolerance by several times. Studies with thoroughbred racing horses and grey-hounds indicated significant reductions in lactic acid buildup, longer endurance, and quicker recovery after racing. Top speed and early top speed was not affected. By improving oxygenation, DMG reduces angina in cardiac patients. Another careful study of fourteen hypertensive patients demonstrated an average drop in diastolic pressure of 14 points (mmHg) over a nine month period. The drop was significant at three months, and continued to decline over the entire period of the trial. The dose used was four tablets per day, which is probably optimal. In that study, cholesterol levels also dropped an average of 12 percent. DMG typically reduces insulin requirements by about 20 percent, and tends to lower blood sugar levels. It typically lowers cholesterol levels, and increases the beneficial HDL levels. It has been proven to prevent posterior subcapsular cataracts in susceptible animals. It has not been proven to reverse PSC cataracts, but appears to do so in early PSC cataracts in my practice. Studies have shown it to dramatically reduce seizures in some epileptics, while they continue to take the supplement.

What is a reasonable dose? An optimal dose would appear to be 125 milligrams sublingually every four hours. That is the amount that prevents (for me) muscle cramping and soreness during strenuous exercise. I do not know what would be an optimal dose without exercise, but the manufacturer recommends 125 to 375 milligrams daily. For patients with PSC cataracts, I am recommending 125 milligrams twice daily in hopes that some benefit will occur, as it frequently does. For patients with angina or out of shape physically, I recommend two tablets (125 milligrams each) prior to exercise, then one tablet every two to four hours during exercise. For diabetics, a trial of two to four tablets per day, while monitoring insulin requirements, is fully justified. Since DMG reduces the incidence of cancer by over 90 percent in susceptible animals (probably due to its production of hydrogen peroxide and immune enhancing properties), it is recommended that persons with cancer take at least two to four tablets per day. This is a non-toxic adjunct to therapy that although has not been proven to be effective in man, has sufficient merit for trial. Any non-toxic substance that has even theoretical benefits is justified when faced with a fatal disease.

Let me share some personal stories. During August of 1986 I began on a jogging program to build my endurance prior to an upcoming Boy Scout hike on the Appalachian Trail. Not having exercised strenuously for several months, my legs began to cramp the first day after 90 seconds (don't laugh, your's will too if you aren't exercising regularly). The second day saw me jog for three minutes before muscle cramping. On the third day I began the use of DMG, 250 milligrams prior to exercise. That day I jogged fifteen minutes without pain, stopping because of a medical emergency requiring my returning to my office. The fourth day I ran 24 minutes, stopping for the same reason, just as I jogged 35 minutes on the fifth day, again being interrupted by a medical emergency. The sixth day (Saturday), I jogged for a full sixty minutes, then went downstairs and bench pressed 75 pounds fifty times (to which I was totally unaccustomed). All without pain, without soreness, and without exhaustion. Nor was I sore the next day. However, I did note some symptoms similar to hypoglycemia, which were relieved by two glasses of juice, making me wonder whether DMG would allow a person to drive himself into severe hypoglycemia. A few weeks later, during the second day of hiking on the Appalachian Trail, my right leg began to cramp about three hours into the hike. That day was mostly climb, mostly above 5,000 foot elevation. I took two magnesium and potassium aspartate tablets (which tends to relax muscle), plus two tablets of DMG. Within a few minutes the cramping left, and I continued to hike another ten hours that day. Again, mostly uphill, and without further soreness. I slept with no discomfort, and hiked the next day refreshed.

The end of September, 1986, I spent the weekend with Gary Null, a talk show host in NYC. Sunday, he ran in the preliminary marathon, and took a large quantity of DMG prior to and during the run. When he returned a few hours later, he was drenched with sweat, but apparently not in the least exhausted. We talked for a while, he took a shower, put on his suit, and went to work. Anyone who knows anything about marathons knows how impressive this is.

I had become a severe diabetic in March of 1986 when I developed the flu and it apparently affected my pancreas. After I found a stable insulin dose, I tried DMG, and it dropped my insulin dose about 20 percent. I have used DMG during strenuous exercise on several other occasions, each time with the same beneficial effect. I have shared this with other "old men" along on the outing, and they, too, did amazingly well. DMG, in my mind, belongs in the home of everyone, especially those of us who have sedentary jobs and work hard on weekends.

A second miracle nutrient is Coenzyme Q10. This also is a naturally occurring enzyme, found in metabolically active tissues such as heart muscle, kidney, liver and pancreas. Vegetable sources of Coenzyme Q10 include spinach (the best source), wheat germ, and most whole grain cereals. Sardines are an impressive dietary source. The best sources we feed to our animals. The "10" refers to the number of groups of identical molecular subgroups attached in chainlike fashion as part of the molecule. Humans need only the Q10 form, but we can convert the other forms to the Q10 type.

We are able to synthesize Coenzyme Q10 when our diet includes adequate amounts of selenium (almost never) and vitamin E (also rare). CoQ10 levels within the body typically decrease with age, and is thought to be one reason why aging and the deterioration of the immune system occurs with years. CoQ10 acts as part of the

Krebs cycle, the basic energy producing metabolic cycle. Thus a deficiency in CoQ10 will result in impaired energy production, and lack of energy. And since every cell in your body requires energy to function, any lack of energy will result your being less than alive.

The heart uses a tremendous amount of energy since it must beat regularly without rest. Cardiac biopsies of persons with heart disease have typically shown CoQ10 deficiencies. More importantly, administration of CoQ10 to persons with heart failure has produced reversal of failure, and with persons suffering acute cardiac infarction (a heart attack) it demonstrably reduces the amount of heart muscle that ultimately dies. In a double blind study of patients with angina, there was a 53 percent reduction in the frequency of angina (heart pain), and an increase in exercise tolerance before onset of angina. According to an article in the *American Journal of Cardiology* (1985;56:247-251) it should be considered a safe and effective treatment for angina.

In studies with patients with congestive heart failure over half of the patients had objective evidence of improvement. Importantly, CoQ10 was able to counteract the toxic side effects of beta blockers (a type of medication used to treat hypertension) without reducing the beneficial effects. Similar beneficial effects were demonstrated with thirty-four patients with severe cardiomyopathy (basically a sick heart). Eighty-two percent improved, and two-year survival rates improved from 25 percent to 62 percent. In other words, their chance of living another two years was more than doubled. Cardiac performance in children with mitral valve prolapse improved in 100 percent of those treated, against no improvement in those on the placebo.

In another study, fifty-four percent of hyptertensives exhibited more than a 10 percent drop in blood pressures after 4-12 weeks of therapy. Seldom was there any drop in pressure prior to four weeks. Interestingly, the beta blocker type of anti-hypertensive drugs tend to inhibit the action of CoQ10, possibly explaining the cardiac toxicity of these drugs. Patients given CoQ10 along with their beta blocker medications did not have the fatigue and malaise side effects of the control group which did not have the CoQ10. In other words, patients who are taking beta blocker medications should also be taking CoQ10 supplements. And may be able to discontinue their anti-hypertensive medications as a result.

Coenzyme Q10 has been proven to reduce fasting blood sugar levels in the majority of diabetics. The drop was as high as 30 percent in 31 percent of those treated. Since CoQ10 is intimately involved in carbohydrate metabolism this perhaps should have been anticipated. From a personal point of view, I was able to reduce my insulin dose within three weeks of taking CoQ10. But, do not stop your insulin without the full knowledge and support of your physician.

Periodontal disease afflicts perhaps 60 percent of young adults, and 90 percent of adults over the age of sixty-five. Coenzyme Q10 deficiency has been demonstrated in various studies in between 60 percent and 96 percent of those with periodontal disease. More importantly, 100 percent of those with periodontal disease not only improved upon administration of CoQ10, but improved with remarkable rapidity. As an aside, rinsing the mouth with a Water-Pik™ using a 3:1 mixture of water and 3 percent hydrogen peroxide produces the same benefit.

Coenzyme Q10 enhances the immune system, perhaps indirectly through the production of DMG, and thereby may be explained the benefit of improved longevity, which is up to 50 percent in animal studies. It also enhances the healing of gastric ulcers. In the animal studies, healing of gastric ulcers was slowed in hypoxic (low oxygen) conditions, and this effect was eliminated through the use of Coenzyme Q10. Again, this effect might be through the production of N,N Dimethylglycine which releases oxygen at the tissue level.

A rather dramatic benefit of Coenzyme Q10 has been demonstrated in treatment of obesity. About 50 percent of obese persons are deficient in this enzyme. When CoQ10 is taken, those who were deficient have a rather dramatic loss of weight. This effect is thought to be due to the enhanced ability to burn calories and more efficient use of oxygen. This enhanced ability to use energy may be one reason why administration of CoQ10 improved work performance even without exercise. Again, it may take a month before benefits manifest. Similarly, we should not be surprised that half of muscular dystrophy patients exhibit subjective and objective improvement upon administration of CoQ10.

Coenzyme Q10 is a potent anti-oxidant, and as with other anti-oxidants tends to reduce aging (it appears to actually reverse aging). It also appears to reduce the severity of allergic reactions in animals, and may be useful in treatment of hay fever and asthma.

It is so effective in treatment of so many diseases that the FDA will make this a prescription drug by the end of 1987. It will continue to be available as an over the counter supplement according to my contact in the FDA.

There is sufficient experimental data to support the use of CoQ10 in the treatment of cardiovascular disease (including congestive heart failure, mitral valve prolapse, angina pectoris, and cardiomyopathy), hypertension, diabetes mellitus (close supervision is essential!), and periodontal disease. Its safety and possible effectiveness suggest its use as an adjunct in ulcer therapy, muscular dystrophy, cancer, and in management of obesity.

Within the past month I have begun to try it with eye patients. One patient with cystoid macular edema unresponsive to everything I could do (including evaluation for laser therapy) for over five years has responded within two weeks with a 60 percent improvement in vision. My own personal effect was a dramatic lowering of my need for insulin, a weight loss of about 8 pounds, and the dramatic appearance of becoming much younger. It is not all appearance, for my ability to focus at near has also improved by several diopters. This appearance of age reversal is proven to happen in animals, and its administration to animals prolongs lifespan by as much as 50 percent, with minimal aging until shortly before death. Another patient of mine, a very intelligent lady who has been unable to lose weight even on a severely restricted diet, lost eighteen pounds the first two weeks of therapy (which was used for an eye condition—which also improved). She had lost eight inches from around her waist in just two weeks. This may be fluid loss from improved kidney function: I certainly lost a lot of fluid during my first week of Coenzyme Q10 therapy.

CoQ10 is virtually non-toxic. It does accumulate in the body, and it would appear that if you are deficient a reasonable dose would be to take about 3,000 milligrams over about three week's time. If you feel a beneficial effect (it may be dramatic), then continue taking 30 milligrams per day. That should saturate your system with the enzyme. To date, no serious adverse effects have been noted. Since it is a food product, and is extremely non-toxic, it should remain available as a non-prescription supplement. Apparently, if you are not deficient it will have no effect, neither toxic nor beneficial. However, it is difficult to obtain more than 3 milligrams per day in the diet (unless you eat sweet meats—kidney, pancreas, liver, heart—regularly). It would appear then that about 10 milligrams per day would be ideal. The gelatin capsule containing pure CoQ10 is the preferred dosage form. The powder has virtually no taste, and has a bright orange color. The product should be labelled as pure Coenzyme Q10. Adulterated products are on the market and use similar, but different, names. The product I use can be obtained through Bio-Zoe, Inc., P.O. Box 49, Waynesville, NC 28786-0049.

A third miracle nutrient is 35 percent food grade hydrogen

peroxide. *However, unlike the two discussed above, hydrogen peroxide is definitely toxic, especially in the 35 percent concentration, and must be used with caution and intelligence.* Food grade hydrogen peroxide is used in the food processing industry to protect packaged foods from growing potentially lethal botulism bacteria. Concentrations of less than 35 percent deteriorate very quickly, and must have additives to stabilize them. These additives are potentially toxic, especially when taken internally. The over-the-counter 3 percent hydrogen peroxide is safe for external use, and even for gargling when diluted, but cannot be taken internally without ill effect.

Therefore, let me caution the reader again that the information given here should not be used without the assistance and knowledge of your physician, preferably one knowledgable in nutritional therapy. Although the benefits seem great, the risks are also great, and you truly venture into uncharted territory.

Those physicians now using hydrogen peroxide in their practice seem to believe that the hydrogen peroxide works by oxygenating the body. And that may be the case. The body produces hydrogen peroxide normally, some of which is used to oxygenate local tissues, and some of which is used to kill invading bacteria. The body has efficient enzymes to neutralize hydrogen peroxide (catalase), and these enzymes are necessary to prevent severe damage from the hydrogen peroxide. The next time you cut yourself, apply some hydrogen peroxide to the wound. The vigorous bubbling that occurs is due to the action of catalase on the hydrogen peroxide, releasing oxygen and water. The point being made is that hydrogen peroxide is not a material foreign to the body, and the body is very well equipped to deal with it.

If you are taking additional hydrogen peroxide, your body naturally will produce more of the enzymes needed. One of the enzymes necessary to deal with the effect of hydrogen peroxide is superoxide dismutase (SOD). I believe that ingestion of hydrogen peroxide forces the body to produce more of this essential SOD. That is speculation. However, it is not speculation that hyperbaric oxygen causes the body to produce more SOD, and that this effect is beneficial. The effect of hydrogen peroxide should be identical to hyperbaric oxygen. (I was the director of hyperbaric medical research with the U.S. Navy at one time, and speak with some authority.) SOD has several beneficial effects, the result of its ability to neutralize free radicals and prolong life. In other words, I believe the beneficial effects of ingested hydrogen peroxide, which have been documented, are the result of improved levels of SOD. If hydrogen peroxide is to boost levels of SOD, the body must have the basic building blocks to make SOD, and these are selenium, zinc, copper, and manganese. As noted elsewhere in this book, selenium and manganese are typically deficient in the majority of Americans, and zinc and copper are frequently deficient.

Hydrogen peroxide is present in fresh fruit and vegetables, rain, spring, and well water in concentrations similar to those used therapeutically. It is not present in canned or cooked fruit and vegetables, nor processed water (all municipal water supplies in the USA). One or two drops in frozen orange juice will result in its tasting like freshly squeezed juice. European cities wisely use hydrogen peroxide to purify their city water supplies—it is far less toxic than chlorine—and may actually be beneficial. Hydrogen peroxide naturally occurs in all water exposed to oxygen or to ultraviolet light. The ozone that gives the clean smell after a thunderstorm reacts with water to form hydrogen peroxide. This concentration of hydrogen peroxide in fresh water, fruit, and vegetables may explain why these foods have been used successfully in treatment of so many diseases, including cancer. Catalyst water, whether generated by the Rockland catalyst device or other means, contains natural levels of hydrogen peroxide. Catalyst water has been used successfully for decades in treatment of degenerative diseases.

In any case, I personally know of patients with terminal cancer (not being treated by me) whose cancer has gone into remission after a few months of ingesting hydrogen peroxide. I also have a patient who on her own had gone on this mode of therapy, and whose hands were virtually useless from arthritis. Within six months her hands looked almost normal, and were fully functional. I know of another lady, again not a patient of mine, whose cataract went away from similar therapy, the remission being affirmed by her ophthalmologist. (Hydrogen peroxide levels within the eye are higher in patients with cataracts. Since hydrogen peroxide is being used to sterilize soft contact lens, and since this cannot be totally removed, there is growing concern that this may produce cataracts. I don't believe this is a problem when the body has adequate levels of zinc, copper, manganese and selenium. But that is unlikely unless you take supplements.) Thus for whatever reason, whether oxygenation or SOD enhancement, hydrogen peroxide ingestion seems to improve health. Again, assuming adequate mineral levels.

I need to emphasize again that 35 percent food grade hydrogen peroxide is highly toxic in its concentrated form. It will burn the skin when applied directly, and probably would prove lethal if ingested without dilution. It has so much oxygen that it will support combustion.

Only the food grade product should be used. It should be transferred to a dark brown glass bottle with a dropper for convenience. Wash your hands and the bottle immediately after use, to prevent bleaching the skin from contact (however, my experience is that this bleaching lasts only about an hour). Hydrogen peroxide *must* be stored safely away from children and infirm adults.

Use *one drop* per glass of liquid the first day, and if you have no toxic effect (nausea), increase this to two drops the next day. Continue until you reach about 3 drops per glass of liquid, or 24 drops per day. *Do not push it to the point that you taste the hydrogen peroxide, nor to the point of nausea.* These symptoms indicate you have overwhelmed your defense systems and may be suffering toxicity. Used properly, hydrogen peroxide represents a homeopathic type therapy. That is, treatment with minute doses of a toxic substance to improve the body's immune system. This is not unlike the use of desensitizing shots used in treatment of allergies. Obviously, you should be tested for adequate levels of selenium, zinc, copper, and manganese (hair analysis recommended), and aggressively treated if these minerals are deficient. I certainly do not recommend use of hydrogen peroxide, although it appears safe as indicated, without assuring myself that these mineral levels are adequate within the body, or therapeutic doses of these elements are concurrently taken.

The maximum dose of 4 drops per glass of liquid would supply 0.03 percent concentration of hydrogen peroxide, which is very quickly decomposed by enzymes within the body.

A scientific article soon to be released by the Bradford Institute strongly urges against use of oral or intravenous hydrogen peroxide. In doses slightly higher than I have recommended here they have demonstrated, or have found literature which demonstrated, that severe toxic effects are occurring by long-term hydrogen peroxide use. Since hydrogen peroxide forms toxic free radicals, they make the logical argument that its use is illogical, especially since we have too many free radicals as it is. Of what value, they say, is it to force the body to produce additional glutathione peroxidase to protect itself? And this is indeed a question which should be answered by carefully monitored studies, not by everyone dosing themselves with a toxic substance.

Whereas I firmly believe that it is fully justified to use non-toxic substances (or doses) such as vitamins in an effort to modify the course of disease, it is not justified to use a toxic substance (such as hydrogen peroxide) without some sort of controlled studies. Since it

214

is obvious that anecdotal evidence exists for beneficial effect, such studies should be funded and undertaken promptly. Until then, my advice will be to avoid use of hydrogen peroxide (except externally), especially avoiding the use of more than 3 drops (of 35 percent) per glass of liquid ingested.

My personal experience is that four drops per glass is hardly noticed, except slightly by taste. Six drops is very noticeable. One day I drank two quarts of water during a meal (I had been working outside), and added four drops per glass. I noticed absolutely no adverse side effects. I did have one very temporary effect: my blood sugar dropped from about 330 to 75 in spite of the meal. (This was during the period of my diabetes.) I have never tried this again to see if it would have the same result. It might actually have been fatal.

Of the supplements discussed in this chapter, all three naturally occur in nature, and in natural foods. Two, N,N Dimethylglycine and Coenzyme Q10, are almost totally non-toxic, it being virtually impossible to ingest toxic quantities. These two have proven benefits. The third, hydrogen peroxide, is also a naturally occurring substance, and appears in the experience of many to reverse many degenerative diseases, perhaps directly (as claimed by some proponents), or perhaps indirectly by inducing production of SOD (which is known to have these benefits) and glutathione peroxidase (also a very beneficial enzyme). This third supplement is very toxic, and must be taken cautiously, in dilute form only, and you must allow your body time to adjust to the dose. Which it will if your body levels of selenium, zinc, copper, and manganese are adequate, which is seldom the case. Because of its potential for harm, I must urge the reader to know his body well and proceed with extreme caution. I would suggest that intermittent use of hydrogen peroxide would be far safer, with probably equivalent benefits, than daily use. However, let the reader beware, for if the cautions by the Bradford Institute are correct, then the potential for harm is great. Indeed, extremely great. I have included this information because I believe it will prove very beneficial in future therapy, once we learn how to use it safely and effectively. I take absolutely no responsibility for misuse of this information. But I am pointing out that many are currently using a toxic substance in doses already proven to be harmful, and this information needs to be spread abroad as quickly as possible.

There is a safe and tested alternative to homebrew hydrogen peroxide. The Rockland Corporation has recently marketed Oxytoddy™, a stabilized mixture of food grade hydrogen peroxide (0.7%), aloe vera juice, and trace mineral concentrates from Body Toddy™. This formula was developed by Dr. Kurt Donsbach over the past several years, and has been used safely with thousands of persons. Since the essential minerals are supplied with the product, and since it is stabilized, it is a logical product for oxygenating the body. According to Dr. Donsbach, maximum benefits are achieved over a six week period. Oxytoddy™ comes in two flavors, cranberry-apple, and herbal tea. Both are very pleasant and leave no unpleasant aftertaste. Oxytoddy™ should be taken on an empty stomach (at least three hours after the last meal), and no food should be consumed for at least thirty minutes after consumption. This is most easily achieved by taking two ounces immediately upon arising, and again immediately before retiring for the evening.

XXIX.
The Body Electric

With apologies to Dr. Robert O. Becker, MD, the author of *The Body Electric*, I have borrowed his catchy title for this chapter. But the use is appropriate: it is the electrical nature of the body which makes the topics discussed herein work, even though we do not understand them. In this chapter, I will be discussing diagnostic techniques currently performed by some physicians, with excellent results. Please use this information cautiously until it is further understood. Nevertheless, these phenomena are of immense importance and relevance; you need very much to be aware of them. For some unknown reason, these techniques do not work for everyone. This is no more understood than why they work for some. The principles involved seem to be the same as in water dousing. If you don't know what that is, ask an oldtimer.

Have someone stand before you with their non-dominant arm (usually the left) extended. Have them remove their watch and set it aside. Tell them that you are going to pull down on their arm, and they are to resist you. Do it. Now place a packet of sugar (such as used in restaurants) in their non-dominant hand, and repeat. Almost invariably, they will be *much* weaker.

Now, have them hold a vitamin E capsule in their dominant hand, while continuing to hold the sugar in their left hand. This time their strength will return, unless they are allergic to vitamin E. Try this with other substances. Toxic substances will produce weakness, beneficial substances will produce increased strength.

Now, set the sugar aside. Have them hold an electronic watch in their hand, and repeat the test. They will be invariably weakened. A self-winding watch will not produce the same effect.

The assumed explanation is that all matter has with it an associated energy field, and this field oscillates at a peculiar frequency. If the energy field of a substance (e.g., sugar) conflicts with your personal energy field, then it weakens you. If it reinforces your energy field, you are strengthened.

This test is called the *kinesiology test*. With it, some physicians are determining whether specific medications are beneficial or

217

harmful, and at what dosage. They claim good results. I am not sufficiently experienced in the art to make a statement, but I do know that there is an instrument approved for medical use in Germany which purports to measure the energy fields in question, and has impressive results.

Another test, used in China for many centuries, works apparently on the same principle. In this test one takes a piece of string with a small object attached in the dominant hand (right hand), and holds the herb or medicine in the palm of the other hand. The object on the string is dangled over the other palm about halfway between the two hands. If the object being tested is beneficial, the string will begin to swing clockwise (supposedly, it will swing in the opposite direction in the southern hemisphere, but I cannot vouch for it). If the object is harmful, it will swing counterclockwise. If neutral, it either will not swing, or will swing back and forth.

Supposedly, the string must not be silk or wool. Supposedly also, the object dangling on the string must contain some metal. That is not true: I found that quartz and cubic zirconium work well. So does a small iron nail; and that seems to work better if it is magnetized. A polyester thread or nylon fishing string works fine.

Sugar usually gives a strong negative reaction. I was showing this to some friends at a covered dish supper, and when I held it over chocolate cake and ice cream, it swung strongly positively for me. For my friend's wife, it practically launched into a counter-clockwise frenzy. She is violently allergic to chocolate. She had not been told in advance what it might do, and in fact it did absolutely nothing when she had held it just moments before over the pie she was eating. Two herbal teas and a decaffeinated tea reacted positively for me. Coffee reacted strongly negatively. Up to 2,000 milligrams of vitamin C usually reacts positively for me, more reacts negatively.

When I use this device, it appears that the nail is being deflected by some sort of force field between my two hands. This deflection is distinct, and easily seen. Again, it doesn't work for everyone. It works best when the testing object (the one on the string) is about half-way between the two hands. If it is an electrical flow of energy, then it would appear that the flow is one way when the object being tested is harmful, another way when it is beneficial. This interpretation is reinforced by the fact that the deflection is stronger when the testing object is magnetized. Quartz, also effective, has a strong associated electrical energy field.

About two years ago, I visited Chief Two Trees and his wife tested me with a device they had. It measured the voltage on each side of each finger, which she wrote down on a chart. She then looked up data in a chart and said that I had a problem with my right rib cage. I did: I had had a rib surgically removed in 1965. She said that I had something wrong with my right kidney. Again right: I had had part of the kidney removed surgically. She said that I had something wrong with my pancreas. "Wrong," I said. Well, about a year later my diabetes became manifest. So she was right, after all. She was right on two other counts. More interestingly, she had never seen me before, and knew nothing about me. I have seen this done, with similar results, on other persons. More sophisticated devices exist and are being used.

I have no doubt that such possibilities lend themselves to charlatans and fraud. But the existence of these energy fields cannot be denied, for they can be both photographed and measured. We must learn what they are, and how they affect us. If Dr. Becker is right, constant exposure to negative force fields can produce degenerative diseases, even cancer. And he has good statistical data to prove it. If an electronic watch weakens a person, does it increase his chances of a heart attack? We need to know. The same goes for magnetic fields from electronic equipment: the epidemic of heart disease coincided with the advent of high powered electronic equipment, and has decreased with the switch to low powered transistor items. Coincidence? We need to know.

I strongly urge you to read Dr. Becker's book *The Body Electric* and come to realize what might be happening. There are constant electrical fields to which we are exposed which might be harmful. Whereas American (USA) standards allow a fairly high level of electromagnetic radiation, Soviet law is far more conservative, and apparently with good reason.

A recent issue of the *Journal of Orthopedics* interviewed an orthopedic surgeon who was actively using pulsed low-energy electromagnetic radiation in treatment of bone injuries. He predicted that within the next decade it will be possible to regenerate amputated limbs (arms and legs). This is in total agreement with Dr. Becker's work. Dr. Becker was even able to prove that regeneration of a severed spinal cord is possible. I have an electromagnetic pulsing device for personal use, and can vouch for the fact that it dramatically speeds healing after surgery or injury. For example, I had injured my right thumb in a skiing accident in January, and by mid-March my thumb was still too sensitive to pick up a glass of water (I had to eat and drink left handed). Five minutes of pulsed radiation relieved the pain to the degree that I could hold a bowl of food, supported entirely by the thumb, with no pain. Although still tender, the original pain has not returned. A friend of mine, who had suffered multiple wrist fractures in an industrial accident, and could not support his hand without a splint, even six months later, was able to remove the splint within two days of treatment.

The original question remains: if these energy fields affect us in such profound ways, what are we doing to ourselves with the high levels of electromagnetic radiation produced in our highly industrialized society? And how could they be modified to produce beneficial effects?

XXX.
To Kill a Child

Ignorance of the law is no excuse in a court of law. When a manufacturer of baby foods a few years back omitted chloride from the foods, many children were permanently brain-damaged, and many died. Ignorance did not defend them from legal repercussions and severe financial losses.

Selenium is essential for healthy hearts. In a controlled study involving 99 percent of children in four communes, China was able to prove that the reason 1.35 percent of their children were dying was selenium deficiency. That is, selenium deficiency was killing four out of every three hundred children. The effects of administering selenium were so dramatic that the placebos were stopped in two years, and by the third year the death rate due to heart disease had dropped to zero. China now adds selenium to their salt as we add iodine. Selenium deficiency has long been known to cause mulberry heart disease in swine, and a similar heart disease in sheep.

Yet, none of the infant formula products I have seen contain any selenium. Obviously, the milk of a nursing mother deficient in selenium will be deficient. But to make a total diet substitute totally devoid of an essential mineral borders on criminal behavior. Yet I do not blame the manufacturers, and I am sure their oversight is unintentional. Their formulas are approved by the American Academy of Pediatrics.

Chromium is also essential for synthesis of heart muscle. It is essential for insulin function. Chromium deficient persons develop hypoglycemia, diabetes, and atherosclerosis, depending on the severity of the deficiency.

Again, none of the infant formulas have even a small amount of this essential mineral. None. Zero. Since most children begin life deficient in chromium (and selenium) because their mothers are deficient, we are allowing our infants to be killed by starvation. And those who survive have crippled immune and enzyme systems that set them up for early degenerative diseases. It is no wonder that in our small county of 45,000 we have had about one teenager per year die of a heart attack. The children don't have a chance, given the ignorance of the medical professional in matters nutritional.

The percentage of calories from fat in the products reviewed (five brands at our local store) was over 45 percent. This is typical of the average American diet, but far higher than the 25 percent recommended by the National Academy of Sciences. Perhaps children require more fat than adults, since cell walls are made of fat. But I don't think they need this much fat. The labels do not indicate the full breakdown of fat types, but indicate only linoleic acid, an essential fatty acid. Do they contain alpha linoleic acid also? The label doesn't say, but I surely hope so.

The formulas appear to be severely deficient in certain vitamins when one compares them to a 2,000 calories adult diet. I suspect that a rapidly growing infant needs at least 50 percent more per calorie than the adult. These include folic acid (essential for growth), biotin (about one-third the minimum amount needed) manganese (less than 1 percent of the amount needed), and magnesium (about 25 percent of the amount needed). If one considers the fact that the RDA is probably far too low for some of these vitamins, one would have to include vitamin C, E, and all of the B vitamins. Copper seems to be about right, except that the high zinc levels probably prevent its absorption.

Several minerals are being supplied in potentially toxic doses. The amount of zinc seems to be high by about 30 percent, and iron is twice what it should be if sufficient vitamin C had been included in the formulas. (Vitamin C enhances iron absorption.).

Some formulas do not include inositol, an essential nutrient. One did include lecithin, from which inositol can be derived. Since deficiencies of these accessory nutrients produce impaired immune systems for life, the cost of misery and health care dollars may be immense.

Ten thousand infants die annually in the USA from sudden infant death syndrome: SIDS. Dr. Archie Kalokerinos of Australia became suspicious when 50 percent of Aborigine children died of SIDS, many within hours of being given a routine DPT injection. In his book *Every Second Child*, he was able to prove without question that vitamin C deficiency was the cause of SIDS. The relationship to a DPT shot becomes obvious when we realize that vitamin C demands soar upon assault on the immune system by viral infection or immunization. Dr. William Torch of the University of Nevada School of Medicine has shown that two-thirds of children dying of SIDS had a DPT shot within three weeks of death, many dying within a day of the immunization. More recent studies in the USA have confirmed the association of immunization with SIDS. The late Dr. Frederick

222

Klenner of Reidsville, NC, was able to reduce the incidence of SIDS among his patients to zero by administering vitamin C to pregnant and nursing mothers.

In other words, 10,000 infants a year are needlessly dying in the USA because their diets do not contain sufficient vitamin C for growth and immune response. The commercial infant formulas contain more than the RDA, but probably should contain at a minimum three times as much for optimal health.

Not only do the commercial infant formulas contain inadequate amounts of many essential minerals, but they are often in forms that are poorly absorbed. The better easily-absorbed forms are considerably more expensive. The high amount of zinc (equivalent to 150 milligrams) found in these formulas will probably block the absorption of copper. Copper is essential to formation of healthy bones and connective tissue (which holds everything together.)

What is the solution? The obvious solution is for mothers to nurse their children the way God intended, and to eat a nutritious and balanced diet, and take supplements when indicated. Supplements recommended include minerals, B-complex, vitamin E, vitamin A, and vitamin C.

The manufacturers of these formulas need to immediately upgrade their formulas to include those minerals and nutrients known to be essential for growth, and mothers need to supplement their children's diet with those minerals and vitamins. This can be done by adding 200 to 400 IU of vitamin E per week to the diet, increasing the vitamin C by the use of buffered powders about 50 milligrams per day (this would be a few granules of powder per day), adding about 200 micrograms of selenium and chromium *per week* by crushing a tablet and adding it to the formula (for the minerals, double this dose for each week old the child is for as many weeks to catch up.) Also add about one-half magnesium-aspartate tablet to the formula every other day. To much magnesium will have a laxative effect. A product such as Bio-Strath™ can be added about 0.5cc (use a dropper) per bottle to supply vitamins and minerals in biologically active forms. These products are available through health food stores everywhere.

The addition of this chapter is a "stop-the-presses" effort. I was unaware of how severely deficient the infant formulas were until a few weeks ago. When I remembered that the USA has the highest infant mortality rate of any civilized nation, and looked at the catastrophe we are bringing upon ourselves, I was aghast. This is a problem that demands immediate attention, and any informed source with reliable suggestions should come forward. Children are dying. They may be yours.

Suggestions for Further Reading

It is not to the credit of my profession that we are so late in discovering that nutrition is one key to healing. However, even that changes, albeit so slowly. When the medical profession finally discovers nutrition you will see advances in preventive health care the likes of which have never before occurred.

The following list is by no means exhaustive, nor complete. It is intended simply to get you started in a study which hopefully will open your life to better health. Just as no one will agree with everything I have said in this book, I do not accept without reservation everything written in these books. It is hoped that by the use of an inquiring mind and common sense that enough good can be gleaned to make your efforts worthwhile.

Airola, Paavo, Ph.D., N.D. *How to Get Well: A Handbook of Natural Healing.* 1974, Health Plus, Publishers, P.O. Box 22001, Phoenix, AZ 85028.

Becker, Robert O., M.D., and Selden, Gary. *The Body Electric: Electro-magnetism and the Foundation of Life,* published by William Morrow & Company, Inc., 1985, New York. $17.95

Bricklin, Mark. *The Practical Encyclopedia of Natural Healing.* (1976, Rodale Press, Emmaus, PA 18049.

Cranton, Elmer M., M.D., and Brecher, Arline. *Bypassing Bypass.* 1984, Stein and Day, Publishers, Scarborough House, Briarcliff Manor, NY 10510. I recommend this as the best available book on chelation therapy (written to a layman), and on free radical pathology.

Gerras, Charles, ed., with the staff of *Prevention* magazine. *The Complete Book of Vitamins.* 1977, Rodale Press, Emmaus, PA 18049.

Isenberg, Seymour, M.D. *Miracle MFM For Fast Weight Loss.* 1983, Executive Reports Corporation, Englewood Cliffs, NJ 07632.

Keough, Carol, ed. *Natural Relief for Arthritis.* 1983, Rodale Press, Emmaus, PA 18049.

Kharasch, Norman, ed. *Trace Metals in Health and Disease.* 1979, Raven Press, 1140 Avenue of the Americas, New York, NY 10036.

Kunin, Richard A., M.D. *Mega-Nutrition: The New Prescription for Maximum Health, Energy, and Longevity.* 1980, McGraw-Hill Book Company, 1221 Avenue of the Americas, New York, NY 10020.

Langer, Stephen E., M.D., and Scheer, James F. *Solved: The Riddle of Illness*. 1984, Keats Publishing, Inc., 27 Pine Street, New Canaan, CT 06840. This book is a very thorough and readable book on hypothyroidism. I urge every physician and intelligent reader to buy and study this book. The information in it is vital to good health.

Lovelock, Jim E. *Gaia: A New Look at Life on Earth*. 1979, The Oxford University Press, Walton Street, Oxford OX2 6DP.

Moore, Richard D. M.D., Ph.D., and Webb, George D., Ph.D.: *The K Factor, Reversing and Preventing High Blood Pressure without drugs*, The MacMillan Publishing Company, NYC, 1986, $17.95.

Ott, John N. *Light, Radiation, and You*. 1982, The Devin-Adair Company, 143 Sound Beach Avenue, Old Greenwich, CT 06870.

Passwater, Richard A., and Cranton, Elmer M., M.D. *Trace Elements, Hair Analysis and Nutrition*. 1983, Keats Publishing Company, Inc., 27 Pine Street, P.O. Box 876, New Canaan, CT 06840. Highly recommended as the definitive work on hair analysis.

Pauling, Linus, Ph.D. *Vitamin C, the Common Cold, and the FLu*. 1976, W. H. Freeman, 41 Madison Avenue, New York, NY 10010.

Pearson, Durk and Shaw, Sandy. *Life Extension: A Practical Scientific Approach*. 1982, Warner Books, 75 Rockefeller Plaza, New York, NY 10019. This book has an extensive bibliography.

Price, Weston A., DDS. *Nutrition and Physical Degeneration*. 1970, Price-Pottenger Foundation, 2901 Wilshire Boulevard, Suite 345, Santa Monica, CA 90403. This book is priceless.

Seelig, Mildred S., M.D. *Magnesium Deficiency in the Pathogenesis of Disease*. 1980, Plenum Publishing, 227 West 17th Street, New York, NY 10011. This is the definitive work on magnesium metabolism.

Shute, Wilfrid E., M.D. *Health Preserver: Defining the Versatility of Vitamin E*. 1977, Rodale Press, Emmaus, PA.

Shute, Wilfrid E., M.D. *Vitamin E for Ailing and Healthy Hearts*. 1972, Pyramid.

Walker, Morton, DPM, and Gordon, Garry, M.D. *The Chelation Answer*. 1982, M. Evans & Co., 216 E. 49th Street, New York, NY 10017.

Index

In Memoriam

*In loving memory of my father,
Joseph Archer Todd, Sr., a loving husband
and father, an accomplished civil engineer,
an author of some rather remarkable poetry
which is only now coming to light.
Born April 11, 1915; returned to the
Lord November 15, 1987.*

The Forgotten Grave

A lonely grave upon a hill
Where sunny summacs grow.
Sunk into the ground and often filled
with water from the rain and snow.
Marked with native rubble stones,
One at head and one at feet.
Chiseled epitaph nearly gone,
Except one line, my love asleep.
No one knows of deeds you did,
Or of trails you might have trod.
From modern man your secrets hid,
But not from almighty God.
No one knows when you died,
Or by whom you were begotten.
No one knows who might have cried,
Only that your grave's forgotten.

—Joe A. Todd